T0226913

Disorders of the Distal Radius Ulnar Joint and Their Surgical Management

Guest Editors

STEVEN L. MORAN, MD
RICHARD A. BERGER, MD, PhD

HAND CLINICS

www.hand.theclinics.com

November 2010 • Volume 26 • Number 4

SAUNDERS an imprint of ELSEVIER, Inc.

W.B. SAUNDERS COMPANY
A Division of Elsevier Inc.

1600 John F. Kennedy Blvd. • Suite 1800 • Philadelphia, Pennsylvania 19103

http://www.theclinics.com

HAND CLINICS Volume 26, Number 4
November 2010 ISSN 0749-0712, ISBN-13: 978-1-4377-2455-4

Editor: Debora Dellapena

© **2010 Elsevier Inc. All rights reserved.**

This journal and the individual contributions contained in it are protected under copyright by Elsevier, and the following terms and conditions apply to their use:

Photocopying
Single photocopies of single articles may be made for personal use as allowed by national copyright laws. Permission of the Publisher and payment of a fee is required for all other photocopying, including multiple or systematic copying, copying for advertising or promotional purposes, resale, and all forms of document delivery. Special rates are available for educational institutions that wish to make photocopies for non-profit educational classroom use. For information on how to seek permission visit www.elsevier.com/permissions or call: (+44) 1865 843830 (UK)/(+1) 215 239 3804 (USA).

Derivative Works
Subscribers may reproduce tables of contents or prepare lists of articles including abstracts for internal circulation within their institutions. Permission of the Publisher is required for resale or distribution outside the institution. Permission of the Publisher is required for all other derivative works, including compilations and translations (please consult www.elsevier.com/permissions).

Electronic Storage or Usage
Permission of the Publisher is required to store or use electronically any material contained in this journal, including any article or part of an article (please consult www.elsevier.com/permissions). Except as outlined above, no part of this publication may be reproduced, stored in a retrieval system or transmitted in any form or by any means, electronic, mechanical, photocopying, recording or otherwise, without prior written permission of the Publisher.

Notice
No responsibility is assumed by the Publisher for any injury and/or damage to persons or property as a matter of products liability, negligence or otherwise, or from any use or operation of any methods, products, instructions or ideas contained in the material herein. Because of rapid advances in the medical sciences, in particular, independent verification of diagnoses and drug dosages should be made.

Although all advertising material is expected to conform to ethical (medical) standards, inclusion in this publication does not constitute a guarantee or endorsement of the quality or value of such product or of the claims made of it by its manufacturer.

Hand Clinics (ISSN 0749-0712) is published quarterly by Elsevier Inc., 360 Park Avenue South, New York, NY 10010-1710. Months of publication are February, May, August, and November. Business and Editorial Offices: 1600 John F. Kennedy Blvd., Ste. 1800, Philadelphia, PA 19103-2899. Customer Service Office: 3251 Riverport Lane, Maryland Heights, MO 63043. Periodicals postage paid at New York, NY and at additional mailing offices. Subscription price is $338.00 per year (domestic individuals), $540.00 per year (domestic institutions), $169.00 per year (domestic students/residents), $385.00 per year (Canadian individuals), $617.00 per year (Canadian institutions), $459.00 per year (international individuals), $617.00 per year (international institutions), and $223.00 per year (international and Canadian students/residents). Foreign air speed delivery is included in all *Clinics* subscription prices. All prices are subject to change without notice. **POSTMASTER:** Send address changes to *Hand Clinics*, Elsevier Health Sciences Division, Subscription Customer Service, 3251 Riverport Lane, Maryland Heights, MO 63043. Customer Service (orders, claims, online, change of address): Elsevier Health Sciences Division, Subscription Customer Service, 3251 Riverport Lane, Maryland Heights, MO 63043. Tel: 1-800-654-2452 (U.S. and Canada); 314-447-8871 (outside U.S. and Canada). Fax: 314-447-8029. E-mail: journalscustomerservice-usa@elsevier.com (for print support); journalsonlinesupport-usa@elsevier.com (for online support).

Reprints. For copies of 100 or more of articles in this publication, please contact the Commercial Reprints Department, Elsevier Inc., 360 Park Avenue South, New York, New York 10010-1710. Tel.: 212-633-3812; Fax: 212-462-1935; E-mail: reprints@elsevier.com.

Hand Clinics is covered in *MEDLINE/PubMed (Index Medicus), Current Contents/Clinical Medicine, EMBASE/Excerpta Medica,* and *ISI/BIOMED.*

Printed and bound by CPI Group (UK) Ltd, Croydon, CR0 4YY

Transferred to Digital Print 2011

Contributors

GUEST EDITORS

STEVEN L. MORAN, MD
Professor and Chair of Plastic Surgery, Division of Plastic Surgery; Associate Professor of Orthopedics, Division of Hand and Microsurgery, Department of Orthopedic Surgery, Mayo Clinic, Rochester, Minnesota

RICHARD A. BERGER, MD, PhD
Professor of Orthopedic Surgery and Anatomy, Mayo Clinic, Rochester, Minnesota

AUTHORS

JULIE E. ADAMS, MD
Assistant Professor, Department of Orthopedic Surgery, University of Minnesota, Minneapolis, Minnesota

KIMBERLY K. AMRAMI, MD
Professor of Orthopedics, Department of Radiology, Chair, Division of Body Magnetic Resonance Imaging, Mayo Clinic, Rochester, Minnesota

RICHARD A. BERGER, MD, PhD
Professor of Orthopedic Surgery and Anatomy, Mayo Clinic, Rochester, Minnesota

BRIAN T. CARLSEN, MD
Assistant Professor, Division of Plastic Surgery, Department of Surgery; Division of Hand Surgery, Department of Orthopaedic Surgery, Mayo Clinic, Rochester, Minnesota

DAVID G. DENNISON, MD
Assistant Professor of Orthopaedic Surgery, Division of Hand Surgery, Department of Orthopaedic Surgery, Mayo Clinic, Rochester, Minnesota

ERIC C. EHMAN, BS
Mayo Medical School, Rochester, Minnesota

BASSEM T. ELHASSAN, MD
Assistant Professor, Department of Orthopedic Surgery, Mayo Clinic, Rochester, Minnesota

JOEL P. FELMLEE, PhD
Professor of Radiologic Physics, Department of Radiology, Mayo Clinic, Rochester, Minnesota

MARC GARCIA-ELIAS, MD, PhD
Consultant, Hand Surgery, Institut Kaplan, Barcelona, Spain

CARL-GÖRAN HAGERT, MD, PhD
Former Willie White Professor, Division of Plastic Surgery, University of Pittsburgh Medical Center, Pittsburgh, Pennsylvania

ELISABET HAGERT, MD, PhD
Consultant Hand Surgeon, Department of Molecular Medicine and Surgery, Section of Orthopaedics, Karolinska Institutet, Stockholm, Sweden

MICHAEL J. HAYTON, FRCS (Tr and Ortho), FFSEM(UK)
Upper Limb Unit, Wrightington Hospital, Wigan, United Kingdom

GUILLAUME HERZBERG, MD, PhD
Professor and Chief, Division of Hand and Upper Extremity Orthopaedic Surgery, Herriot Hospital and Claude Bernard University, Lyon, France

SANJEEV KAKAR, MD, MRCS, MBA
Assistant Professor, Division of Hand Surgery, Department of Orthopaedic Surgery, Mayo Clinic, Rochester, Minnesota

RUDY KOVACHEVICH, MD
Resident, Department of Orthopedic Surgery,
Mayo Clinic, Rochester, Minnesota

ALBERTO LLUCH, MD, PhD
Associate Professor of Orthopaedic Surgery;
Orthopaedic and Hand Surgeon, Institut
Kaplan for Surgery of the Hand and Upper
Extremity, Barcelona, Spain

STEVEN L. MORAN, MD
Professor and Chair of Plastic Surgery, Division
of Plastic Surgery; Associate Professor of
Orthopedics, Division of Hand and
Microsurgery, Department of Orthopedic
Surgery, Mayo Clinic, Rochester,
Minnesota

A. LEE OSTERMAN, MD
Professor of Orthopedic Surgery, Philadelphia
Hand Center, Thomas Jefferson University,
King of Prussia, Pennsylvania

WENDY L. PARKER, MD, PhD
Assistant Professor, Department of Surgery
Scott and White Clinic, Texas A&M University,
Temple, Texas

TAMIR PRITSCH, MD
Hand Fellow, Department of Orthopedics,
Mayo Clinic, Rochester, Minnesota

MARCO RIZZO, MD
Associate Professor and Consultant,
Division of Hand Surgery, Department
of Orthopedic Surgery, Mayo Clinic,
Rochester, Minnesota

DOUGLAS M. SAMMER, MD
Assistant Professor of Surgery, Division
of Plastic Surgery, Washington University
School of Medicine, St Louis, Missouri

JOHN K. STANLEY, FRCS, FRCSEd
Upper Limb Unit, Wrightington Hospital,
Wigan, United Kingdom

SCOTT P. STEINMANN, MD
Professor, Department of Orthopedic
Surgery, Mayo Clinic, Rochester,
Minnesota

SHIAN-CHAO TAY, MD, MS
Assistant Professor of Orthopedic Surgery,
Mayo Clinic, Rochester, Minnesota; Assistant
Professor of Hand Surgery, Singapore General
Hospital, Singapore

ADAM C. WATTS, FRCS (Tr and Ortho)
Upper Limb Unit, Wrightington Hospital,
Wigan, United Kingdom

Contents

The authors describe the anatomy of the distal radioulnar joint (DRUJ) and delineate the importance of viewing this joint as part of the whole forearm. The osseous congruity and ligamentous integrity is of essence for the stability of the DRUJ, according to the principles of tensegrity. The neuromuscular control and possible proprioceptive function of the DRUJ are also outlined.

Imaging the DRUJ requires knowledge of the complex bony, muscular, and ligamentous anatomy that contribute to this unique joint. Standard well-positioned radiography is always the appropriate first step in any imaging evaluation of the wrist. High-resolution MRI of the wrist, preferably performed at 3T, helps to delineate the important ligamentous structures relevant to the DRUJ and ulnar wrist, whether the joint is unstable or not. The presence of instability on physical examination is an indication for dynamic CT evaluation. Close attention to technique, no matter what the modality of choice, offers the best chance for success in providing added value with imaging. Finally, communication between the radiologist and hand surgeon allows the advanced imaging examinations to be tailored to the specific clinical problem for the most effective use of resources for each individual patient.

For the distal radioulnar joint (DRUJ) to be stable, not only do the articulating surfaces need to be congruent and well aligned but also the capsule and ligaments need to be mechanically and sensorially competent. According to recent investigations, ligaments should not be regarded as simple static structures maintaining articular alignment but as complex arrangements of collagen fibers containing mechanoreceptors, which are able to generate neural reflexes aiming at a more efficient and a more definitive muscular stabilization. By careful planning and meticulous execution of surgical incisions to approach the DRUJ, the nerve endings innervating the capsule and DRUJ ligaments may be safeguarded, thus preserving the proprioceptive function of the joint.

Injury to the triangular fibrocartilage complex is the most common cause of ulnar-sided wrist pain. This functionally related complex of anatomic structures can be a source of pain secondary to acute injury or chronic degeneration. Strategies for the treatment of these injuries involve determining the anatomic location of the tear, the presence of associated distal radioulnar joint instability, and the presence of associated degenerative changes. Surgical management with open and arthroscopic techniques have been described, both with successful results.

Unlike tears of the peripheral triangular fibrocartilage or avulsions of the distal radioulnar ligaments, longitudinal split tears of the ulnotriquetral (UT) ligament do not cause any instability to the distal radioulnar joint or the ulnocarpal articulation. It is mainly a pain syndrome that can be incapacitating. However, because the UT ligament arises from the palmar radioulnar ligament of the triangular fibrocartilage complex (TFCC), it is by definition, an injury of the TFCC. The purpose of this article is to describe the cause of chronic ulnar wrist pain arising from a longitudinal split tear of the UT ligament.

This article reviews acute dislocations of the distal radioulnar joint (DRUJ) and distal ulna fractures. Acute dislocations can occur in isolation or in association with a fracture to the distal radius, radial metadiaphysis (Galeazzi fracture), or radial head (Essex-Lopresti injury). Distal ulna fractures may occur in isolation or in combination with a distal radius fracture. Both injury patterns are associated with high energy. Outcomes are predicated on anatomic reduction and restoration of the stability of the DRUJ.

The stabilizing constraints of the distal radioulnar joint (DRUJ) include its bony geometry and the surrounding soft tissue support. Given the shallow nature of the sigmoid notch, reconstruction of the palmar and dorsal ligamentous sleeve provides the best solution for restoring stability in cases of chronic DRUJ instability. The pertinent anatomy, indications, contraindications, soft tissue stabilizing procedures, and rehabilitation for the management of chronic DRUJ instability are highlighted in this review.

In the patient in whom primary distal radioulnar joint surgery has failed, consideration must be given to the anatomy and biomechanics of the native joint; how this has been disrupted by injury, disease, and previous trauma; and what is required to reconstruct the joint. The forearm relies on a congruent condylar cam of the distal ulna, with intact soft tissue restraints for normal biomechanics. Surgical reconstruction using tendon graft, autologous bone graft, allograft interposition, and prosthetic reconstruction are discussed in this article. If these procedures fail, then salvage procedures including wide excision of the ulna or one-bone forearm can be performed.

Injury to the interosseous membrane of the forearm typically occurs in conjunction with disruption of the radial head and the distal radioulnar joint. Frequently, the true extent of injury is not initially appreciated, and patients may develop longitudinal instability of the forearm, with wrist pain, forearm discomfort, and instability. This article outlines various treatment strategies, which include considerations at the wrist, forearm, and elbow.

Ulnar impaction syndrome is a common source of ulnar-sided wrist pain. It is a degenerative condition that occurs secondary to excessive load across the ulnocarpal joint, resulting in a spectrum of pathologic changes and symptoms. It may occur in any wrist but is usually associated with positive ulnar variance, whether congenital or acquired. The diagnosis of ulnar impaction syndrome is made by clinical examination and is supported by radiographic studies. Surgery is indicated if nonoperative treatment fails. Although a number of alternatives exist, the 2 primary surgical options are ulnar-shortening osteotomy or partial resection of the distal dome of the ulna (wafer procedure). This article discusses the etiology of ulnar impaction syndrome, and its diagnosis and treatment.

Arthrodesis is the most reliable and durable surgical procedure for the treatment of a joint disorder, with the main disadvantage of loss of motion of the fused joint. The distal radioulnar joint can be arthrodesed, while forearm pronation and supination are maintained or even improved by creating a pseudoarthrosis of the ulna just proximal to the arthrodesis. This is known as the Sauvé-Kapandji procedure. This procedure is not void of possible complications, such as nonunion or delayed union of the arthrodesis, fibrous or osseous union at the pseudoarthrosis, and painful instability at the proximal ulna stump. All of these can be prevented if a careful surgical technique is used.

Metallic ulnar head implants have been proposed not only to solve symptomatic radioulnar impingement after Darrach or Sauvé-Kapandji procedures, but also to prevent such an impingement when treating arthritic distal radioulnar joint. This article prospectively analyzes a series of ulnar head implants with special reference to bone resorption at the prosthesis collar and erosion of the sigmoid notch of the distal radius at an average follow-up of 32 months (minimum 24 months).

Pain in the ulnar aspect of the pediatric wrist is an uncommon problem; however, when pain does occur it is usually the result of antecedent bony trauma or an underlying skeletal abnormality, which may lead to ulnar-sided wrist pain of varying etiology. The clinician must to be able to identify these entities within the pediatric wrist in order to make the appropriate diagnosis and plan for surgical intervention to prevent ongoing damage to the distal radioulnar joint (DRUJ). This article reviews the etiology, clinical presentation, and treatment strategies for the management of the unique problems that can affect the pediatric and adolescent DRUJ.

Hand Clinics

THE CLINICS ARE NOW AVAILABLE ONLINE!

Access your subscription at:
www.theclinics.com

Preface

Disorders of the Distal Radius Ulnar Joint and Their Surgical Management

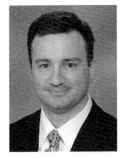 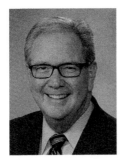

Steven L. Moran, MD   Richard A. Berger, MD, PhD
Guest Editors

In 1998 Dr Thomas Graham edited an issue of the *Hand Clinics* entitled "Problems About the Distal End of the Ulna"; that issue of the *Hand Clinics* remained on my desk for the better part of three years as I kept returning to it for clarification on the anatomy, biomechanics, and the pathophysiology of the distal radial ulnar joint (DRUJ). Since that time, the DRUJ has remained an area of discovery and controversy within the field of hand surgery. The complexity of diagnoses within this area and the lack of established treatment algorithms have led my coeditor, Dr Richard Berger, to occasionally refer to the management of these problems as "DRUJury." Fortunately, recent advancements in imaging and arthroscopy have allowed hand surgeons to identify injuries in this area earlier, while continued anatomic research has allowed for the development of improved surgical approaches and anatomic reconstructions of some DRUJ injuries.

Within this issue of *Hand Clinics*, we have enlisted the help of some of the pioneers in field of DRUJ research, as well as some of the new champions in the field of DRUJ arthroplasty and arthroscopy. In 1998, Dr Graham noted in his preface that "hand surgery requires dedication to life-long learning,"[1] and as a testimony to that statement this issue of *Hand Clinics* is meant to build upon the previous works of Dr Lawrence Schenider in 1991 and Dr Graham in 1998. It is our hope that the questions and controversies elicited within this text will entice another group of hand surgeons to write the 4th "edition" of the *Hand Clinics* devoted to problems of the DRUJ in 10 more years as hand surgeons continue to pursue surgical perfection within the ulnar aspect of the wrist.

My coeditor, Richard Berger, and I would like to thank our esteemed authors who have work so hard to contribute to this text. In addition, we would like to thank Debora Dellapena and the entire editorial staff at Elsevier for their assistance and patience in the completion of this issue of *Hand Clinics*.

Steven L. Moran, MD
Division of Plastic Surgery
Department of Surgery
Division of Hand Surgery
Department of Orthopaedic Surgery
Mayo Clinic
200 First Street SW
Rochester, MN 55905, USA

Richard A. Berger, MD, PhD
Division of Hand Surgery
Department of Orthopaedic Surgery
Mayo Clinic
200 First Street SW
Rochester, MN 55905, USA

E-mail addresses:
moran.steven@mayo.edu (S.L. Moran)
berger.richard@mayo.edu (R.A. Berger)

REFERENCE

1. Graham TJ. Preface. Hand Clin 1998;14(2):154.

doi:10.1016/j.hcl.2010.09.001
0749-0712/10/$ — see front matter © 2010 Elsevier Inc. All rights reserved.

Understanding Stability of the Distal Radioulnar Joint Through an Understanding of Its Anatomy

Elisabet Hagert, MD, PhD[a],*, Carl-Göran Hagert, MD, PhD[b]

KEYWORDS

- Anatomy • Distal radioulnar • Joint
- Joint stability • Proprioception • Wrist

The stability of a joint is primarily dependent on 2 intimately working factors: the congruity of the convex and concave articulating surfaces throughout the range of joint motion, and the static stability of intact joint ligaments.[1] Additionally, there is a secondary dynamic stability from muscles acting to compress the joint.[2] Hence, in the clinical setting of analyzing a patient with joint instability, the following questions must be answered: Are the 2 articulating surfaces congruous? Are the stabilizing ligaments unharmed?

The human distal radioulnar joint (DRUJ) has evolved through time to become, beyond comparison, the most unique articulation in the body. The phylogeny of the DRUJ has moved from being a blocklike construction in 4-legged mammals in need of forward propulsion,[3] to a precise articulation capable of both load bearing and rotation of 160 degrees or more. The evolution of the DRUJ has even been proposed as a key element in the humanoid transition from being a food gatherer to being a food producer.[4]

In the following presentation of DRUJ anatomy, we illuminate 3 views of this complex joint system: (1) anteroposterior (AP) view of the forearm in full pronation, (2) lateral view of the forearm in neutral position, and (3) distal view of the distal radioulnar

(DRU) articulation. The first 2 views are aimed at understanding the osseous anatomy and stability of the DRUJ, whereas the last is aimed at primarily understanding the ligamentous components of stability.

ANTEROPOSTERIOR VIEW OF THE FOREARM IN FULL PRONATION

In the AP view of the forearm, an important aspect of understanding DRUJ anatomy and stability is evident. The DRUJ is not a joint per se, but rather the distal compartment of one joint, the forearm joint, of which the proximal part is the proximal radioulnar joint, the PRUJ.[5]

To illustrate this, let us assume that we make an osteotomy through the radius and the ulna just distal to the PRUJ and, similarly, just proximal to the DRUJ (**Fig. 1**A) and remove the radial and ulnar shafts to apposition the ends of the forearm. Having done that, we will find we have "created" a perfect bicondylar joint with 2 convex articulating surfaces of equal size and 2 concave counterparts, also of equal size (**Fig. 1**B). This bicondylar joint has its axis of rotation through the center of the convex articulating surfaces (the radial and

[a] Karolinska Institutet, Department of Molecular Medicine and Surgery, Section of Orthopaedics, Stockholm, Sweden
[b] Division of Plastic Surgery, University of Pittsburgh Medical Center, PA, USA
* Corresponding author. Hand & Foot Reconstructive Surgery Center, Storangsv.10, Stockholm 115 42, Sweden.
E-mail address: elisabet.hagert@ki.se

Hand Clin 26 (2010) 459–466
doi:10.1016/j.hcl.2010.05.002
0749-0712/10/$ – see front matter © 2010 Published by Elsevier Inc.

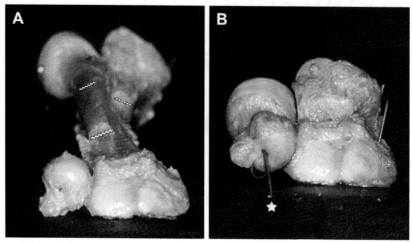

Fig. 1. The forearm joint. (*A*) Distal view of the forearm in pronation. The site of proposed osteotomies are seen as zigzag lines. (*B*) After removal of the shafts in *A*, the proximal and distal ends of the forearm are placed in apposition to reveal the bicondylar forearm joint. *, axis of rotation in the ulnar head. (*Courtesy of* Elisabet Hagert, MD, PhD, Stockholm, Sweden.)

ulnar heads, respectively), which remains unchanged even as we reposition the 2 previously removed shafts to recreate the full forearm in pronation. It should be noted that the forearm joint, even though truly being a bicondylar joint, has a particular shape, whereas the radius has its convex articulating surface proximally (the radial head) but its concave surface (the semilunar notch) distally, and for the ulna, vice versa. This construction enables the pronated forearm to supinate about 160 degrees by a swing of the distal end of the radius around the stable, nonrotating ulnar head.

LATERAL VIEW OF THE DRUJ AND THE WHOLE FOREARM

Because the DRUJ is an articulation at the distal end of the forearm joint, as described previously, it has to be studied both as part of the whole forearm as well as a separate "joint" in itself. Hence, to have a complete clinical and radiographical examination of the DRUJ, the forearm should be positioned as follows:

1. The upper arm in adduction (adjacent to the trunk)
2. The elbow flexed 90 degrees with the forearm in a neutral position (0 degrees pronation/supination)
3. The fingers of the hand in a neutral position and the thumb at the side of the second metacarpal to create a flattened hand with the ulnar side down and the thumb up.

This position is easy to reproduce, as the flattened hand is consistently positioned in the flexion-extension plane of the elbow, and both the forearm and the DRUJ will then, by definition, be in a neutral position.[6] With the patient thus positioned, our clinical examination will be well defined, as we can measure the range of motion in pronation and supination and evaluate the stability both in neutral and in any position of rotation, as well as estimate the strength in pronation and supination using, for instance, a transversely loaded pronosupination test.[7]

In this position, we can also readily understand that the ulnar head is the immobile, nonrotating and weight-bearing part of the forearm, which supports the radius, the hand, and what we hold in the hand.

THE LATERAL VIEW AND RADIOGRAPHIC EXAMINATION OF THE DRUJ

The lateral view and position of the forearm and hand described previously is optimal for the 2 projections required for a complete radiographic assessment of the DRUJ.

- Position 1: With the x-ray beams projected perpendicular to the flexion-extension plane of the elbow, a straight *AP* view of the radius with the radial styloid forming the radial contour, and a straight *lateral* view of the ulna with its styloid forming the ulnar contour, is achieved (**Fig. 2**A).

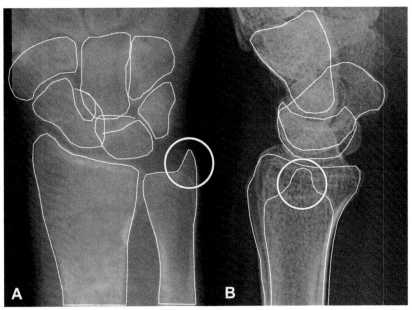

Fig. 2. Radiographic imaging of the DRUJ. (*A*) AP view of the DRUJ will provide a lateral profile of the ulnar styloid (circled), whereas (*B*) a true lateral view of the DRUJ will give an AP view of the ulnar styloid (*circled*).

- Position 2: With the beams coinciding with the flexion-extension plane of the elbow, a straight *lateral* view of the radius and a straight *AP* of the ulna with the styloid shown in the center, is achieved (**Fig. 2**B).

It should be stressed that the forearm shall be maintained in a neutral position throughout the examination, and only the x-ray tube rotated 90 degrees to achieve the 2 necessary projections. Furthermore, although radiographic examinations (including magnetic resonance imaging and computed tomography) are of value in identifying joint incongruency and/or possible ligament injuries, an actual instability of the DRUJ is purely a clinical diagnosis.

DISTAL VIEW OF THE DRUJ

Following exarticulation of the hand at the radio-carpal level, the distal view will show the distal radius with its 2 facets and the triangular-shaped radioulnar ligament (**Fig. 3**). Its central, fibrocartila-ginous and avascular region, the "disc," is in this case resected, leaving the dorsal and volar bundles of the radioulnar ligament exposed. The ligaments emanate from the ulnar-dorsal and ulnar-volar corners of the distal radius, respec-tively, and converge ulnarly to insert primarily into the fovea of the distal ulna, with a portion of the ligaments extending onto the ulnar styloid (**Fig. 4**).[8]

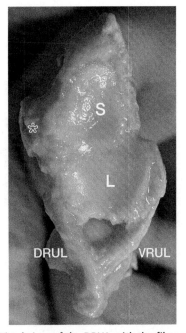

Fig. 3. Distal view of the DRUJ, with the fibrocartilagi-nous portion of the central disc excised. The dorsal radioulnar ligament (DRUL) and volar radioulnar liga-ment (VRUL) are clearly seen emanating from the dorsal and volar ulnar corners of the distal radius, inserting onto the distal ulna. L, lunate facet; S, the scaphoid facet; *, lister's tubercle. (*Courtesy of* Elisa-bet Hagert, MD, PhD, Stockholm, Sweden.)

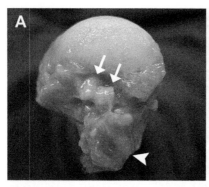
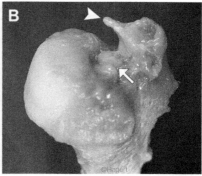

Fig. 4. The insertions of the DRU ligaments onto the ulnar head in (*A*) distal view and (*B*) lateral view. The 2 bundles of the DRU ligaments are clearly seen inserting into the fovea (*arrows*), with a smaller and superficial portion of the ligaments inserting onto the ulnar styloid (*arrowheads*). (*Courtesy of* Elisabet Hagert, MD, PhD, Stockholm, Sweden.)

Akin to the structure of the anterior cruciate ligament (ACL) of the knee,[9] we found in our dissections of the DRUJ that the fibers of the radioulnar ligaments have a spiral rotation upon insertion into the fovea (**Fig. 5**). From studies on the spiral configuration of the ACL, it has been proposed that this will allow different portions of the ACL to be taut, and therefore functional, throughout all ranges of knee motion, engaging various bundles at different joint angles.[10,11]

A similar arrangement may be assumed in the wrist and is described through the following dissections:

As long as the structure of the PRUJ is intact, the radius can be moved into pronation and supination while the radioulnar ligaments are studied. Upon a primary inspection of the DRU ligaments from a distal view, it is evident that in *pronation*, the dorsal radioulnar bundle is taut compared with the volar bundle, which is redundant in character (**Fig. 6**A).

By performing a meticulous layer-by-layer excision of the superficial fibers of the ligaments, there is a shift in constraint properties where the deep volar radioulnar bundle becomes taut, whereas the deep dorsal bundle appears slack (**Fig. 6**B). Apparently, there is a shift in ligamentous tension from a superficial to a deeper layer—fibers that are taut in the superficial layer are slack on the depth, and vice versa. This arrangement was first described through an anatomic publication 15 years ago,[12] and has recently been confirmed in an in vivo kinematic study of the radioulnar ligaments.[13] In general, the deep bundles are found to insert in the fovea as compared with the eccentric and prestyloid insertion of the superficial fibers.[14]

Finally, the dissection is brought to a complete excision of the dorsal bundle, keeping only the volar bundle in place as a thin strand. Despite this rudimentary remnant of the volar radioulnar ligament, the radioulnar congruency is maintained (**Fig. 6**C). Thus, stability of the DRUJ is maintained by 2 factors: compression between the articulating surfaces and tension in the ligament in the direction of its fibers.

TENSEGRITY—THE CORE OF DRUJ STABILITY

Through the aforementioned description of stability, the DRUJ may be understood as a structure of *tensegrity*. The concept of tensegrity was first visualized by sculptor Kenneth Snelson in 1948 (**Fig. 7**) and later defined by architect R. Buckminster Fuller in 1961, as the integrity of structures based on a *synergy of tension and*

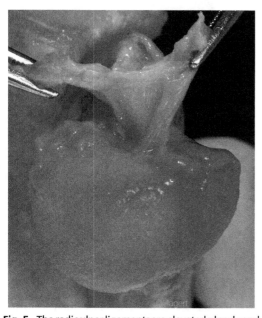

Fig. 5. The radioulnar ligaments are elevated ulnarly and viewed from below. The spiral configuration of the ligaments upon insertion into the fovea is clearly seen. (*Courtesy of* Elisabet Hagert, MD, PhD, Stockholm, Sweden.)

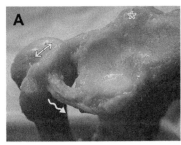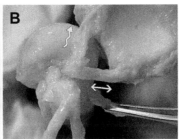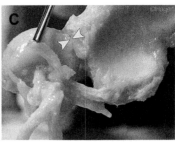

Fig. 6. Understanding the stability of the DRUJ. (*A*) Distal view of the DRUJ in pronation. The DRUL appears taut (*double arrow*) and the volar radioulnar ligament (VRUL) redundant (*curved arrow*). (*B*) Meticulous dissection of the superficial fibers of the ligaments reveals an inverse relationship in the deep fibers, and the DRUL is now slack, whereas the VRUL is taut. (*C*) After complete sectioning of the DRUL, the joint is still congruent. The compression of the dorsal joint surfaces (*arrowheads*) and the tension of the opposing volar ligament maintain the stability of the joint. *, lister's tubercle. (*Courtesy of* Elisabet Hagert, MD, PhD, Stockholm, Sweden.)

compression forces. Fuller writes: "Tension and compression are inseparable and coordinate functions of structural systems… [that] are mechanically stable not because of the strength of individual members but because of the way the entire structure distributes and balances mechanical stresses."[15] The concept of tensegrity has been further integrated into human medicine by Dr D. E. Ingber, who describes in his article, "The Architecture of Life,"[16] how tensegrity is found in all aspects of the human body, from skeleton to cytoskeleton. Ingber further clarifies the concept of tensegrity: "Tensegrity structures…share one critical feature, which is that tension is continuously transmitted across all structural members. In other words…a global increase in tension is balanced by an increase in compression within certain members spaced throughout the structure. In this way, the structure stabilizes itself through a mechanism that Fuller described as continuous tension and local compression." A similar concept of tension and compression as related to hand surgery has previously been described in relation to the anatomy of the metacarpophalangeal joint.[17]

With these definitions in mind, let us look closer at the architecture of the DRUJ.

The curvature of the convex articulating surface of the ulnar head measures about 10 mm in radius with the origin of the bow of the circle at the fovea of the ulnar head (**Fig. 8**). This origin corresponds with the axis of forearm rotation located in the ulnar head, and also the origin of the deep portions of the volar and dorsal DRU ligaments.

The curvature of the semilunar notch measures about 15 mm in radius with the origin positioned near the base of the ulnar styloid. This is an epicentric displacement of approximately 5 mm from the axis of rotation, and corresponds with

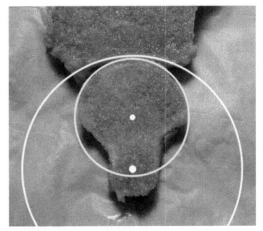

Fig. 8. Transverse section through the distal radius and ulna. The smaller, inner circle depicts the curvature of the ulnar head with its center (*small dot*) equivalent to the region of the fovea. The larger, outer circle illustrates the curvature of the semilunar notch on the distal radius and its center (*large dot*) correlates to the ulnar styloid. (*Courtesy of* Elisabet Hagert, MD, PhD, Stockholm, Sweden.)

Fig. 7. Tensegrity, as depicted in a sculpture by Kenneth Snelson (*Mozart I*, 1982) at Stanford University.

the insertion of the superficial fibers in the prestyloid recess (see **Fig. 8**).

Based on this architectural arrangement, the following is apparent.

The distal end of the radius moves around the fixed ulnar head in terms of a translational movement, not rotational. A translational movement results in continuous changes in the contact areas between the semilunar notch and the ulnar head. At the neutral position, approximately 60% of the cartilage surfaces are in contact, whereas at the extremes of pronosupination only about 10%, corresponding to an area of 1 to 2 mm, are in contact.[18,19]

The radioulnar ligaments have a spiral configuration as they insert into a surface area, not one single point, on the ulnar head. The helicoidal bundles, in conjunction with the combined centric and epicentric insertions of the deep and superficial radioulnar portions, respectively, lead to a continuous shift in the tension of various portions of the ligaments. This continuous shift in tension and compression constitutes the core of DRUJ stability, and is the essence of tensegrity. The stability of the DRUJ is thus a constantly changing and dynamic process, which lends as a conclusion that there is no clinical relevance to discuss which fibers are taut and which are not in any separate position of rotation.

When the forearm is viewed as a whole, a rotation motion (pronosupination) may be understood as the radius moving around the immobile ulna. The proximal radius is performing a strict rotation around an axis positioned in the center of the radial head. The distal radius, however, performs a swing around an axis of rotation positioned about 10 mm medial of the radius, equivalent to the fovea of the ulnar head. Hereby, a full pronosupination motion of the DRUJ entails a translation motion of the concave surface of the semilunar notch toward the convex ulnar head throughout a motion arc of 160 degrees or more, at a distance of 25 cm from its proximal counterpart, the PRUJ. This superb architectural arrangement is, of course, dependent not only on the congruity of the DRUJ, but also on a maintained osseous congruity of the entire forearm.

NEUROMUSCULAR CONTROL OF THE DRUJ

Although the DRUJ is thus a structure of tensegrity, with inherent stability dependent on an osseous and ligamentous integrity and their interplay of tensile and compressive forces, it is secondarily influenced by the dynamic forces acting on the joint. From other joints,[20–23] it is established that the dynamic control of a joint is dependent on its sensorimotor function where afferent information from mechanoreceptors within ligaments or capsules affect the function in the muscles controlling that joint through so-called *proprioception*.[24,25] The details of the neuromuscular control of the DRUJ are at this stage veiled in obscurity, but factors influencing the dynamic stability of the DRUJ are outlined later in this article.

Innervation of the DRUJ and Its Ligaments

Anatomic studies on the innervation of the DRUJ have revealed a threefold pattern, where the dorsal region is primarily innervated by the terminal branch of the posterior interosseous nerve, the ulnar region primarily by the dorsal sensory branch of the ulnar nerve, and the volar region by branches from the ulnar nerve.[26,27] Although branches of the anterior interosseous nerve (AIN) have been shown in the vicinity of the volar DRUJ capsule,[28,29] detailed microscopic studies have not been able to show AIN afferents in the DRUJ ligaments.[26] Similarly, the medial antebrachial cutaneous nerve has an extra-articular course in the DRUJ,[29,30] but lacks intra-articular contributions.[26,31]

Cavalcante and colleagues[32] additionally analyzed the microscopic innervation of the DRU ligaments. Using gold-chloride staining and light microscopy, they were able to identify both slowly and rapidly adapting mechanoreceptors (Pacini corpuscles and Ruffini endings, respectively) as well as free nerve endings, suggesting a proprioceptive function of the DRU ligaments.

Muscular Stability of the DRUJ

Because the DRUJ is the distal half of the forearm joint, any rotation motion of the entire forearm will influence the dynamic stability of the DRUJ. However, the sole contributor to direct muscular stability of the DRUJ is the pronator quadratus (PQ), as its anatomy directly affects the function of the DRUJ (**Fig. 9**). The PQ is consistently found to consist of a superficial and a deep head, which span the distal volar surface of the radius and ulna, just proximal to the DRUJ.[33] In vivo electromyographic analysis of the stabilizing function of the PQ has revealed that the PQ, in particular the

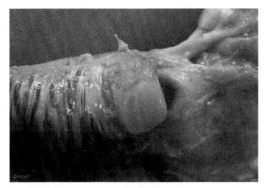

Fig. 9. The intimate relationship of the pronator quadratus muscle to the distal radioulnar joint is seen here, with the muscle enveloping the volar aspect just proximal to the DRUJ. (*Courtesy of* Elisabet Hagert, MD, PhD, Stockholm, Sweden.)

deep head, is active during both pronation and supination of the forearm, suggesting that this muscle has a primary function as a dynamic stabilizer of the DRUJ.[34] The PQ may thus be important in a neuromuscular training of patients with hyperlaxity or subclinical instabilities of the DRUJ.[35]

The extensor carpi ulnaris (ECU) has additionally been proposed to have a stabilizing role of the DRUJ in forearm supination, as the relationship of the tendon sheath to the groove of the ulnar head may resist abnormal displacement of the ulnar head.[36] The ECU has been shown to have a slight torque effect on the DRUJ, with a potential pronation torque in maximal supination and vice versa in pronation.[37] However, in vitro analysis of the direct effect of the ECU and its subsheath on DRUJ translation have not been able to delineate a significant contribution to the stability of the DRUJ, but rather confirmed the importance of the osseous and ligamentous components.[38] However, the true details of the in vivo neuromuscular and proprioceptive functions of the DRUJ remain to be illuminated.

SUMMARY

A thorough appreciation of the anatomy of the distal radioulnar joint is incumbent for an understanding of its stability. The DRUJ should be seen as the distal half of the forearm joint, where any fracture affecting the forearm may affect the stability at the DRUJ. An osseous congruity and ligamentous integrity of the DRUJ is fundamental for the stability of the joint.

ACKNOWLEDGMENTS

We express our sincere gratitude to the Department of Anatomy, Karolinska Institutet, Stockholm, Sweden, in particular to Lars Winblad, without whom these anatomic studies would not have been possible. We are also indebted to Dr Otte Brosjö, Department of Orthopedics, Karolinska University Hospital, Stockholm, Sweden, for assistance in the collection of samples.

REFERENCES

1. Linscheid RL, Dobyns JH, Beabout JW, et al. Traumatic instability of the wrist. Diagnosis, classification, and pathomechanics. J Bone Joint Surg Am 1972;54(8):1612–32.
2. Linscheid RL, Dobyns JH. Dynamic carpal stability. Keio J Med 2002;51(3):140–7.
3. Ladd AL. Upper-limb evolution and development: skeletons in the closet. Congenital anomalies and evolution's template. J Bone Joint Surg Am 2009; 91(Suppl 4):19–25.
4. Almquist EE. Evolution of the distal radioulnar joint. Clin Orthop Relat Res 1992;(275):5–13.
5. Hagert CG. The distal radioulnar joint in relation to the whole forearm. Clin Orthop Relat Res 1992;(275): 56–64.
6. Gilula LA, Mann FA, Dobyns JH, et al. Wrist terminology as defined by the International Wrist Investigators' Workshop (IWIW). J Bone Joint Surg Am 2002;84(Suppl 1):1–66.
7. Garcia-Elias M, Lluch AL, Ferreres A, et al. Transverse loaded pronosupination test. J Hand Surg Eur Vol 2008;33(6):765–7.
8. Garcia-Elias M, Domenech-Mateu JM. The articular disc of the wrist. Limits and relations. Acta Anat (Basel) 1987;128(1):51–4.
9. Girgis FG, Marshall JL, Monajem A. The cruciate ligaments of the knee joint. Anatomical, functional and experimental analysis. Clin Orthop Relat Res 1975;(106):216–31.
10. Mommersteeg TJ, Huiskes R, Blankevoort L, et al. An inverse dynamics modeling approach to determine the restraining function of human knee ligament bundles. J Biomech 1997;30(2):139–46.
11. Sakane M, Fox RJ, Woo SL, et al. In situ forces in the anterior cruciate ligament and its bundles in response to anterior tibial loads. J Orthop Res 1997;15(2):285–93.
12. Hagert CG. Distal radius fracture and the distal radioulnar joint—anatomical considerations. Handchir Mikrochir Plast Chir 1994;26(1):22–6.
13. Xu J, Tang JB. In vivo changes in lengths of the ligaments stabilizing the distal radioulnar joint. J Hand Surg Am 2009;34(1):40–5.
14. Nakamura T, Takayama S, Horiuchi Y, et al. Origins and insertions of the triangular fibrocartilage complex: a histological study. J Hand Surg Br 2001;26(5):446–54.
15. Buckminster Fuller R. Tensegrity. Portfolio and Arts News Annual 1961;4:112–27.

16. Ingber DE. The architecture of life. Sci Am 1998; 278(1):48–57.

17. Hagert CG. Anatomical aspects on the design of metacarpophalangeal implants. Reconstr Surg Traumatol 1981;18:92–110.

18. af Ekenstam F, Hagert CG. Anatomical studies on the geometry and stability of the distal radio ulnar joint. Scand J Plast Reconstr Surg 1985;19(1):17–25.

19. Hagert CG. The distal radioulnar joint. Hand Clin 1987;3(1):41–50.

20. Johansson H, Sjolander P, Sojka P. A sensory role for the cruciate ligaments. Clin Orthop 1991;(268): 161–78.

21. Solomonow M. Sensory-motor control of ligaments and associated neuromuscular disorders. J Electromyogr Kinesiol 2006;16(6):549–67.

22. Hagert E. Wrist ligaments—innervation patterns and ligamento-muscular reflexes [PhD Thesis]. Department of Clinical Science and Education, Section of Hand Surgery, Karolinska Institutet, Stockholm; 2008. p. 1–51.

23. Hagert E, Persson JK, Werner M, et al. Evidence of wrist proprioceptive reflexes elicited after stimulation of the scapholunate interosseous ligament. J Hand Surg Am 2009;34(4):642–51.

24. Lephart SM, Fu FH. Proprioception and neuromuscular control in joint stability. Champaign (IL): Human Kinetics; 2000. p. 1–439.

25. Riemann BL, Lephart SM. The sensorimotor system, part I: the physiologic basis of functional joint stability. J Athl Train 2002;37(1):71–9.

26. Gupta R, Nelson SD, Baker J, et al. The innervation of the triangular fibrocartilage complex: nitric acid maceration rediscovered. Plast Reconstr Surg 2001;107(1):135–9.

27. Shigemitsu T, Tobe M, Mizutani K, et al. Innervation of the triangular fibrocartilage complex of the human wrist: quantitative immunohistochemical study. Anat Sci Int 2007;82(3):127–32.

28. Ferreres A, Suso S, Ordi J, et al. Wrist denervation. Anatomical considerations. J Hand Surg Br 1995; 20(6):761–8.

29. Fukumoto K, Kojima T, Kinoshita Y, et al. An anatomic study of the innervation of the wrist joint and Wilhelm's technique for denervation. J Hand Surg Am 1993;18(3):484–9.

30. Wilhelm A. Zur Innervation der Gelenke der oberen Extremität. [Innervation of the joints of the upper extremity]. Z Anat Entwicklungsgesch 1958;120(5): 331–71 [in German].

31. Ohmori M, Azuma H. Morphology and distribution of nerve endings in the human triangular fibrocartilage complex. J Hand Surg Br 1998;23(4): 522–5.

32. Cavalcante ML, Rodrigues CJ, Mattar R Jr. Mechanoreceptors and nerve endings of the triangular fibrocartilage in the human wrist. J Hand Surg Am 2004;29(3):432–5 [discussion: 436–8].

33. Stuart PR. Pronator quadratus revisited. J Hand Surg Br 1996;21(6):714–22.

34. Gordon KD, Pardo RD, Johnson JA, et al. Electromyographic activity and strength during maximum isometric pronation and supination efforts in healthy adults. J Orthop Res 2004;22(1):208–13.

35. Hagert E. Proprioception of the wrist joint: a review of current concepts and possible implications on the rehabilitation of the wrist. J Hand Ther 2010; 23(1):2–17.

36. Garcia-Elias M. Soft-tissue anatomy and relationships about the distal ulna. Hand Clin 1998;14(2): 165–76.

37. Haugstvedt JR, Berger RA, Berglund LJ. A mechanical study of the moment-forces of the supinators and pronators of the forearm. Acta Orthop Scand 2001;72(6):629–34.

38. Stuart PR, Berger RA, Linscheid RL, et al. The dorsopalmar stability of the distal radioulnar joint. J Hand Surg Am 2000;25(4):689–99.

Imaging the Distal Radioulnar Joint

Kimberly K. Amrami, MD[a,*], Steven L. Moran, MD[b,c],
Richard A. Berger, MD, PhD[d], Eric C. Ehman, BS[e],
Joel P. Felmlee, PhD[a]

KEYWORDS

- DRUJ • Wrist • Triangular fibrocartilage complex
- CT • MRI

Imaging the distal radioulnar joint (DRUJ) represents a unique challenge for radiologists and hand surgeons alike. The joint must be evaluated for static, dynamic, and functional relationships as well as for abnormalities involving the bones, ligaments, and muscles that constitute the DRUJ. A multimodal approach is required in most cases to definitively understand the underlying mechanisms of DRUJ dysfunction.

ANATOMY

The DRUJ consists of a multitude of complex relationships involving the bones, muscles, and ligaments. The articulation of the ulnar head with the distal radius at the sigmoid notch not only allows significant degrees of freedom for pronation and supination but also accommodates distal and proximal translations of the ulna relative to the distal radius, making evaluation of this joint a 3-dimensional exercise. The articular surfaces of the sigmoid notch and ulnar head do not match when viewed axially: the arc of the sigmoid notch is significantly larger than the ulnar head, which accounts for some of its large degrees of freedom and some of its inherent tendency toward instability resulting from its relatively tenuous ligamentous and tendinous constraints. Radiography and computed tomography (CT) are excellent tools for the evaluation of the bony anatomy of the joint.[1–3] In addition to the constraints of the joint itself, there are critical ligamentous structures that help to stabilize the DRUJ. These structures include the palmar and dorsal radioulnar ligaments, the ulnocarpal ligaments, and the triangular fibrocartilage complex (TFCC). The distal radioulnar ligaments are in continuity with the body or disk; the ulnotriquetral ligaments arise from the disk or body of the TFCC. This intimate relationship is evident on sagittal magnetic resonance (MR) images (**Fig. 1**). The attachment of the TFCC to the ulnar fovea (foveal attachment), a critical component of DRUJ stability, is also evident on high-resolution magnetic resonance imaging (MRI).[4,5]

RADIOGRAPHY

Radiography remains the mainstay of all initial evaluations of the hand and wrist, including the DRUJ.[6] Neutral posteroanterior (PA) radiography is helpful for the assessment of degenerative changes of the DRUJ and ulnar variance.[7] Lateral radiography has a special role in assessing the alignment of the unloaded DRUJ. On a well-positioned lateral radiograph, it is possible to assess with a high degree of confidence the relationship of the distal ulna relative to the radius; normal alignment shows overlap of the 2 bones with no dorsal or volar displacement of the ulna. However, this assessment is dependent on accurate positioning of the wrist on the lateral radiograph—more difficult than it seems at first glance. The wrist is commonly positioned on the lateral view in some degree of supination, which confounds the assessment of the relationship of the forearm bones. The accuracy of positioning

[a] Division of Body Magnetic Resonance Imaging, Mayo Clinic, 200 First Street SW, Rochester, MN 55905, USA
[b] Division of Plastic Surgery, Mayo Clinic, 200 First Street SW, Rochester, MN 55905, USA
[c] Department of Orthopedic Surgery, Mayo Clinic, 200 First Street SW, Rochester, MN 55905, USA
[d] Division of Hand Surgery, Mayo Clinic, 200 First Street SW, Rochester, MN 55905, USA
[e] Mayo Medical School, 200 First Street SW, Rochester, MN 55905, USA
* Corresponding author.
E-mail address: amrami.kimberly@mayo.edu

Hand Clin 26 (2010) 467–475
doi:10.1016/j.hcl.2010.07.001
0749-0712/10/$ – see front matter © 2010 Elsevier Inc. All rights reserved.

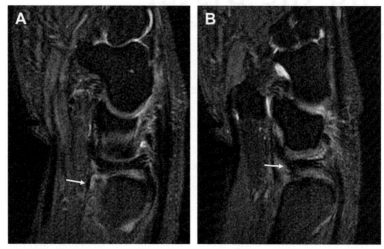

Fig. 1. (*A*) Sagittal T2-weighted fast spin echo (FSE) MR image with fat suppression showing the palmar radioulnar ligament arising from the disk of the TFCC (*arrow*). (*B*) Sagittal T2-weighted FSE MR image with fat suppression showing the origin of the ulnotriquetral ligament from the palmar radioulnar ligament (*arrow*).

can be evaluated by comparing the relative positions of the distal pole of the scaphoid, pisiform, and capitate bones. The distal pole of the scaphoid and pisiform, each representing the most palmar portions of the carpus at its radial and ulnar aspects, can be compared with the palmar cortex of the capitate, which represents a relative midpoint. The pisiform and distal pole of the scaphoid should overlap the palmar cortex of the capitate. The pisiform should be essentially transected in half by the palmar cortex of the capitate, and the anterior cortex of the distal pole of the

scaphoid should not extend beyond the margin of the pisiform (**Fig. 2**). If the pisiform is volar to the anterior cortex of the capitate, the image is supinated, and if it is more dorsally located relative to the anterior cortex of the capitate, the image is pronated. In either case, true alignment of the DRUJ cannot be determined and other relationships, such as the angulation of the distal radius on the lateral view, can be difficult to assess.[6,8,9]

Additional radiographic views, including radial and ulnar deviated PA radiographs and the "motion" series, may be useful for assessing wrist

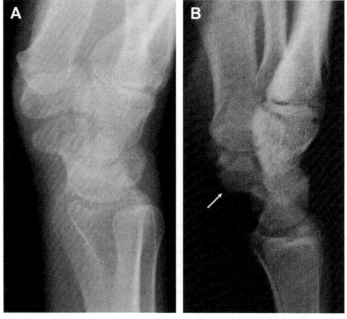

Fig. 2. (*A*) Lateral radiograph of the wrist showing dorsal subluxation of the ulna on a well-positioned image. (*B*) Lateral radiograph of the wrist positioned in supination with underestimation of DRUJ subluxation.

pain but have limited added value for assessing the DRUJ. Fluoroscopic examinations of wrist positioning in real time may help to localize pain, which may occur only under dynamic conditions or with specific types of joint loading.

SCINTIGRAPHY

Scintigraphy has a role in the assessment of the DRUJ when attempting to distinguish the joint itself as a source of ulnar-sided wrist pain, especially when degenerative arthritis may be the cause of pain but radiography is unrevealing (**Fig. 3**). Scintigraphy is also helpful when early inflammatory arthritis is suspected. Single-phase scintigraphy has high sensitivity and specificity for active bone turnover but is nonspecific to identify the underlying cause. Anatomic imaging is almost always required for correlation with the bone scan—it is rarely a stand-alone test. Three-phase bone scans (flow, blood pool, and delayed phases) may be helpful in distinguishing inflammation from infection when used in association with labeled white blood cell imaging, but infection is rarely a concern with the DRUJ. In general, scintigraphy is most helpful when other types of anatomic imaging, such as radiography, MRI, and CT, have shown no abnormality but there is persistent unexplained pain or disability. In that situation, a negative bone scan result is reassuring and a positive bone scan result showing definite activity helps to redirect diagnostic investigations.

CT

CT has become an important part of assessing the DRUJ.[1–3] In addition to its unique ability to depict bony anatomy at very high resolutions without the use of contrast or extended imaging times, it is possible to rapidly image the DRUJ in different loading conditions to assess dynamic displacement in cases in which instability of the DRUJ is suspected clinically. CT cannot demonstrate ligamentous anatomy as effectively as MRI, but the consequences of any ligamentous injuries may be assessed semiquantitatively using positioning with loading and resistance. Historically, patients' wrists were imaged in unloaded conditions in neutral positioning, pronation, and supination, all in the axial plane, to visualize the relationship between the distal radius and ulna at these extremes of the range of motion. This procedure was rarely informative unless the abnormality was obvious. Current approaches focus on imaging the joint in different degrees of loading and resistance to better simulate the physiologic conditions. This can be accomplished in a variety of ways, including using weighted sandbags or other weights that may be either gripped or placed over the hand to increase the force of pronation or supination. Alternatively, as in the authors' practice, a device that provides joint loading via resistance in different degrees of pronation, supination, and neutral positioning can be used. Patients lie prone on the CT table with arms raised over their heads and grip a device that can be set at the neutral position or at 60° of pronation or supination (**Fig. 4**). Patients' wrists are first imaged in the neutral position at each of these stations bilaterally, and then, the patients are asked to actively pronate or supinate against the grip in each position. Axial images only through the DRUJ are taken in each of the positions, for a total of 9 separate sets of images. The images are then assessed

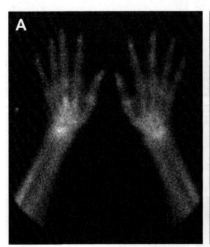
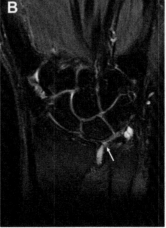

Fig. 3. (*A*) Bone scan from a patient with bilateral ulnar wrist pain showing nonspecific uptake at the radiocarpal joint on each side. (*B*) Coronal T2-weighted fast spin echo MR image with fat suppression showing the synovitis and radial-sided tear (*arrow*) explaining the activity on the bone scan.

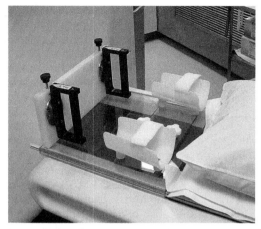

Fig. 4. Device for use with CT for dynamic DRUJ imaging. (*Courtesy* of Richard A. Berger, MD, PhD, Rochester, MN).

visually for displacement of the DRUJ by determining the position of the ulna relative to the radius at the joint. If a foveal tear or tear of the dorsal radioulnar ligaments is the source of the pathologic condition, the examination typically shows the most dorsal displacement of the ulna when the patient performs pronation in the 60° pronation position, with some degree of displacement in all pronation positions on the affected side (**Fig. 5**). Unilateral palmar displacement in the supine or neutral position may be seen in the case in which there is an isolated tear of the palmar radioulnar ligament, but this is rare. Bilateral symmetric

multidirectional displacement of the ulna throughout the range of motion may be seen as a normal variant in individuals with relatively lax joints.

Caution should be exercised in the interpretation of this study to assure correlation with the physical examination. In the authors' practice, the affected joint is injected with an anesthetic before the CT examination so that the strength testing is performed clinically and the examination will not be limited by pain. Performing CT without first addressing pain may lead to underestimation of the degree of displacement, as patients protect their joint against discomfort. Another potential pitfall is the situation in which there is a symmetric dorsal displacement or the unaffected side shows dorsal displacement greater than that seen on the side under investigation. Without the benefit of clinical correlation, this pitfall might result in the overestimation of what may be a normal variation (**Fig. 6**). It is helpful for the radiologist to have the results of the clinical examination available before interpreting the results of CT and all functional radiological examinations.

CT also has a role in assessing the DRUJ anatomically, particularly after trauma to the distal radius that may involve the DRUJ.[10] The articular surface of the distal radius can be evaluated for congruence, and any loose bodies or bone fragments within the joint can be easily seen. The images can be reformatted in multiple planes, and 3-dimensional reformatting is performed to

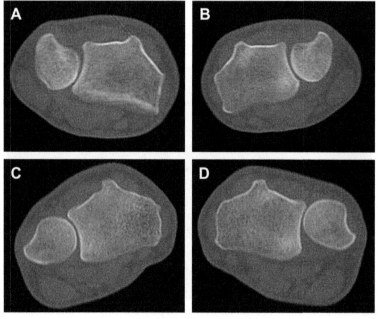

Fig. 5. Patient imaged with dynamic loaded CT in neutral position (*A, B*) and 60° of resisted pronation (*C, D*). Note the dorsal displacement of the ulna on the left in pronation (*D*), corresponding to clinical instability of the DRUJ.

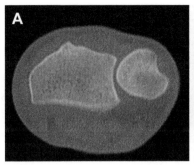
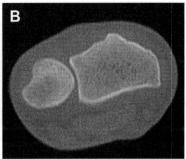

Fig. 6. Axial CT images from a patient with left (*B*) ulnar-sided pain in resisted pronation. Note the dorsal displacement of the ulna on the right (*A*), which is the patient's unaffected side. No instability was present clinically.

even all disarticulation of the joint for visualization of all the joint surfaces before any surgical intervention.

MRI

MRI has become one of the most important tools in diagnosing problems of the DRUJ.[4,5] MRI allows direct visualization of the ligaments associated with the DRUJ, including the palmar and dorsal radioulnar ligaments, the ulnocarpal ligaments, and the TFCC with its critical foveal attachment to the distal ulna. Tears of the palmar and dorsal radioulnar ligaments are relatively rare but can be seen after direct trauma or falls on an outstretched hand; they rarely are a direct cause of DRUJ pain or instability (**Fig. 7**). Tears of the ulnar attachments of the TFCC are much more common and more likely to be a source of pain or instability at the DRUJ, including the styloid or foveal attachments and the ulnocarpal (particularly, the ulnotriquetral) ligaments. With the appropriate MRI technique, which includes high-resolution imaging

and appropriate sequences with a dedicated wrist receiver coil, all these structures can be identified on routine imaging of the wrist. If available, 3-T MRI is preferred, but 1.5-T MRI may be effective with an optimized technique.[4,5,11] In general, low-field open MR scanners are not appropriate for wrist imaging.[4] Recent innovations in dedicated extremity magnets, now available at 1.5 T, show some promise for wrist imaging, which may be a more accessible technology than conventional whole-body MRI. MR arthrography with intra-articular gadolinium is not generally necessary for evaluation of the ulnar wrist and DRUJ.

The foveal attachment is best seen on a combination of coronal and sagittal imaging. A normal TFCC and attachments are low in signal intensity

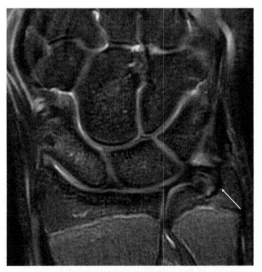

Fig. 8. Coronal T2-weighted fast spin echo image of the wrist with fat suppression showing the normal foveal attachment of the TFCC inserting on the distal ulna (*arrow*).

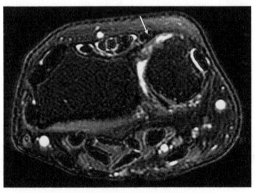

Fig. 7. Axial T2-weighted fast spin echo MR image of the wrist with fat suppression showing a tear of the dorsal radioulnar ligament (*arrow*).

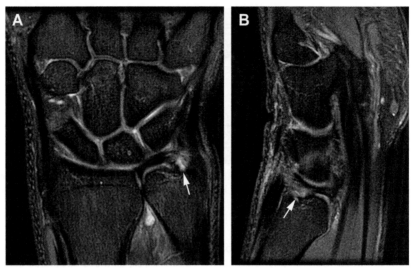

Fig. 9. T2-weighted fast spin echo MR images of the wrist with fat suppression in 2 patients with ulnar-sided wrist pain. (*A*) A high-grade partial tear at the foveal insertion in a patient without DRUJ instability (*arrow*). (*B*) Complete foveal dissociation in a patient with gross instability on examination (*arrow*). Both patients had a positive foveal sign.

on all sequences (the normal appearance of fibrocartilage and ligaments), and the foveal attachment is seen as a direct attachment to the bone (**Fig. 8**). There is a normal synovial reflection at this site, which should not be mistaken for an abnormality in the attachment itself. In the case of a complete tear or disruption, there is usually fluid interposed between the torn attachment and the bone (**Fig. 9**), which is best seen on fluid-sensitive sequences, such as T2-weighted fast spin echo with chemical fat suppression or short time inversion recovery. This is usually associated with clinical instability of the joint either on physical examination or on a dynamic CT study. If the wrist is positioned in pronation with padding the positioning itself acts as some resistance. This results in dorsal displacement of the ulna on the axial images, similar to what is seen on the dynamic CT study (**Fig. 10**). If the fovea is partially torn, some of the fibers should be seen attached to the ulna despite abnormal signal or tearing in the remainder of the attachment. In this situation, the DRUJ is usually clinically stable, and hence, no significant displacement would be expected. It is critical to make this distinction: correlation with physical examinations and findings, such as the "foveal sign" and stability of the DRUJ on physical examination, will help to improve the accuracy and relevance of the imaging assessment.[12]

Complete or partial tears of the fovea rarely occur in isolation. More commonly, they are associated with tears, either partial or complete, of the

ulnotriquetral ligament and the body or disk of the TFCC (**Fig. 11**). Tears of any of these structures may lead to a positive foveal sign and significant pain at the ulnar wrist and DRUJ, but only complete disruption of the foveal attachment is associated with DRUJ instability.[5,12] A well-performed MR examination of the wrist with attention to technique and detail shows all these structures to excellent effect.[4,5]

In addition to the complex ligament tears, which may cause pain and instability at the DRUJ, the joint itself is a source of pain because of either

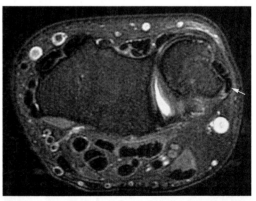

Fig. 10. Axial T2-weighted fast spin echo MR image with fat suppression showing dorsal displacement of the DRUJ with the patient positioned in pronation for the MRI. This patient had a complete foveal tear and an extensor carpi ulnaris (ECU) subsheath tear with subluxation of the ECU (*arrow*).

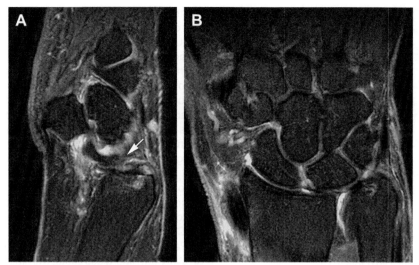

Fig. 11. Sagittal (*A*) and coronal (*B*) T2-weighted fast spin echo MR images of the wrist in a patient with ulnar wrist pain and no instability. There is a partial tear of the ulnotriquetral ligament extending into the foveal attachment, but no complete disruption is present (*arrow*).

degenerative arthritis, usually associated with previous trauma, or malalignment of the joint. Inflammatory arthritis may also affect the DRUJ either primarily or through erosion of the foveal attachment of the TFCC at the distal ulna, a classic finding in early rheumatoid arthritis detected by the consistent synovial reflection at the ulnar fovea. MRI effectively shows chondromalacia, any malunion related to previous fractures, and the extent of synovitis within the DRUJ, radiocarpal joint, and the carpus. Abnormalities in the muscles supporting the DRUJ are unusual, but a muscle tear or strain could theoretically cause pain in or

weakness of the DRUJ. An interesting MRI finding is slight T2 hyperintensity within the pronator quadratus muscle in the normal state, best seen on 3-T MRI. This finding is likely because of the activation of this postural muscle at rest and does not represent any sort of strain or other abnormality within the muscle.

POSTOPERATIVE IMAGING

There are many options available for repair or reconstruction of the DRUJ and its associated ligamentous and muscular structures. In most

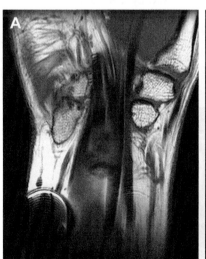
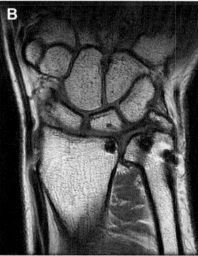

Fig. 12. Coronal T1-weighted fast spin echo MR images of the wrist in 2 patients after DRUJ repair. (*A*) Metallic artifact from a cobalt ulnar head prosthesis, but good visualization of the mid and distal wrist. (*B*) Ligamentous reconstructions with excellent visualization of the tunnels in the radius and ulna with minimal metallic artifact.

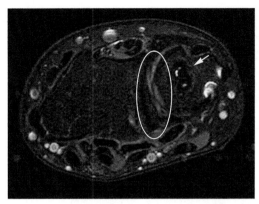

Fig. 13. Axial T2-weighted fast spin echo MR image with fat suppression after DRUJ reconstruction in a patient with recurrent pain after surgery. The graft is intact (*arrow*), but the patient has developed chondromalacia in the DRUJ (*oval*).

cases, postoperative imaging consists of routine PA and lateral radiography to assess relationships among the bones and the integrity of any implant (such as the Berger U-head) or anchor related to ligament repairs (**Fig. 12**). Cross-sectional imaging is not generally indicated for routine follow-up but rather is reserved for problem solving for patients with recurrent pain or instability. CT may be performed to compare relationships among bones before and after surgery, and the same functional study of DRUJ stability using dynamic CT imaging may be performed in patients after surgical intervention. More commonly, MRI is performed to determine whether repairs are intact or whether tears have recurred in patients with pain and/or instability after surgical intervention. In most cases, the area where surgery was performed has some metallic artifact from the instrumentation used, from implants, or from sutures; the effect of these metallic artifacts can be greatly diminished

by the use of advanced MRI techniques. Although the overall image quality is somewhat affected, the DRUJ itself and the TFCC and its ligamentous attachments should be visible. Reconstructions of the DRUJ with muscle division and tendon repositioning through tunnels in the radius and ulna can also be seen and continuity of the grafts assessed. In addition to assessing the integrity of the repairs, it is also possible to diagnose other sources of pain at the DRUJ, which may be unrelated to the surgery, such as the development of arthritis in the joint (**Fig. 13**). Postoperative imaging may also show successful restoration of the normal alignment of the DRUJ in pronation secondary to reconstruction of the foveal attachment of the TFCC (**Fig. 14**).

Patients' wrists may be imaged with CT and MRI in short-arm fiberglass casts, with little or no artifact related to the cast itself (**Fig. 15**). Image quality may be slightly compromised on MRI because of the need for a larger receiver coil to accommodate the cast, but the diagnostic value of the scan is not inhibited in most cases.

IMAGING ALGORITHM

Imaging the DRUJ always begins with PA and lateral radiography, with special attention to positioning the lateral view. If further imaging is needed, the choice of the next test depends on the findings on the physical examination. In most cases in which clinical instability is present, a dynamic CT study to assess the degree of ulnar displacement and asymmetry with the unaffected side is helpful for decision making before surgery, followed by MRI to determine the exact point of ligamentous disruption. If clinical instability is not present, the CT study is unlikely to be revealing and MRI is suggested as the appropriate next test. Postoperative imaging usually involves MRI unless the question is specifically regarding

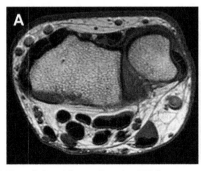
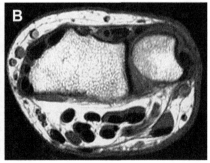

Fig. 14. Axial T1-weighted fast spin echo MR images with the patient imaged in pronation before (*A*) and after (*B*) repair of foveal and subsheath tears of the TFCC. Note the normalization in the postoperative image (*B*) of the alignment of the DRUJ.

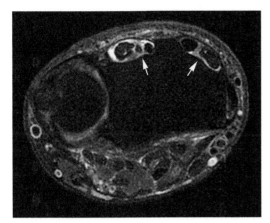

Fig. 15. Axial T2-weighted fast spin echo image with fat suppression obtained with a patient in a cast after TFCC repair. Note the extensor tenosynovitis of the second, third, and fourth extensor compartments (*arrow*).

congruity of the DRUJ after trauma, in which case a CT with multiplanar reformatting is the most helpful test.

SUMMARY

Imaging the DRUJ requires knowledge of the complex bony, muscular, and ligamentous anatomy that contribute to this unique joint. Standard well-positioned radiography is always the appropriate first step in any imaging evaluation of the wrist. High-resolution MRI of the wrist, preferably performed at 3 T, helps to delineate the important ligamentous structures relevant to the DRUJ and ulnar wrist, whether the joint is unstable or not. The presence of instability on physical examination is an indication for dynamic CT evaluation. Close attention to technique, no matter what the modality of choice, offers the best chance for success in providing added value with imaging. Finally, communication between the radiologist and hand surgeon allows the advanced imaging examinations to be tailored to the specific clinical problem for the most effective use of resources for each individual patient.

REFERENCES

1. Tay SC, Berger RA, Tomita K, et al. In vivo three-dimensional displacement of the distal radioulnar joint during resisted forearm rotation. J Hand Surg Am 2007;32:450–8.
2. Nakamura R, Horii E, Imaeda T, et al. Criteria for diagnosing distal radioulnar joint subluxation by computed tomography. Skeletal Radiol 1996;25: 649–53.
3. Mino DE, Palmer AK, Levinsohn EM. The role of radiography and computerized tomography in the diagnosis of subluxation and dislocation of the distal radioulnar joint. J Hand Surg Am 1983;8:23–31.
4. Amrami K. Radiology corner: basic principles of MRI for hand surgeons. J Am Soc Surg Hand 2005;5: 81–6.
5. Amrami KK, Felmee JP. 3-Tesla imaging of the wrist and hand: techniques and applications. Semin Musculoskelet Radiol 2008;12:223–37.
6. Amrami KK, Berger RA. Radiology corner: review of plain radiographs. J Am Soc Surg Hand 2005;5: 4–7.
7. Levis CM, Yang Z, Gilula LA. Validation of the extensor carpi ulnaris groove as a predictor for the recognition of standard posteroanterior radiographs of the wrist. J Hand Surg Am 2002;27:252–7.
8. Kumar A, Iqbal MJ. Missed isolated volar dislocation of distal radio-ulnar joint: a case report. J Emerg Med 1999;17:873–5.
9. Zanetti M, Gilula LA, Jacob HA, et al. Palmar tilt of the distal radius: influence of off-lateral projection—initial observations. Radiology 2001;220: 594–600.
10. Mulford JS, Axelrod TS. Traumatic injuries of the distal radioulnar joint. Hand Clin 2010;26:155–63.
11. Anderson ML, Skinner JA, Felmlee JP, et al. Diagnostic comparison of 1.5 Tesla and 3.0 Tesla preoperative MRI of the wrist in patients with ulnar-sided wrist pain. J Hand Surg Am 2008;33:1153–9.
12. Tay SC, Tomita K, Berger RA. The "ulnar fovea sign" for defining ulnar wrist pain: an analysis of sensitivity and specificity. J Hand Surg Am 2007; 32:438–44.

REFERENCES

Surgical Approaches to the Distal Radioulnar Joint

Marc Garcia-Elias, MD, PhD[a],*, Elisabet Hagert, MD, PhD[b]

KEYWORDS

- Distal radioulnar joint • Proprioception
- Surgical approaches • Triangular fibrocartilage complex

For the distal radioulnar joint (DRUJ) to be stable, not only do the articulating surfaces need to be congruent and well aligned but also the capsule and ligaments need to be mechanically and sensorially competent. According to recent investigations, ligaments should not be regarded as simple static structures maintaining articular alignment but as complex arrangements of collagen fibers containing mechanoreceptors, which are able to generate neural reflexes aiming at a more efficient and a more definitive muscular stabilization.[1–4] It is certainly through a proper interaction of the 2 major DRUJ constraints, namely the triangular fibrocartilage (TFC) and the ulnocarpal ligaments, and the 2 most effective DRUJ muscle stabilizers, the extensor carpi ulnaris (ECU) and the pronator quadratus (PQ) muscles, that joint stability is achieved.[5–7] Indeed, patients with substantial passive laxity of the DRUJ may remain asymptomatic if the destabilizing forces experienced by the joint are anticipated and quickly inhibited by an adequate ECU and PQ muscle reaction. If the time between aggression and muscle reaction, the so-called latency time, is unusually prolonged, instability may worsen and result in further ligament injury.[1,2] The latency time, however, is directly dependent on the speed of afferent proprioceptive stimuli from the mechanoreceptors in the joint to the spinal cord, and back to the muscles. If the DRUJ capsule and ligaments have been denervated, muscle reactions may also appear, but the response may not be quick enough to provide stability, because this neuromuscular reaction will be a result of afferent stimuli from extra-articular receptors in adjacent tendons and skin. Joint denervation, a procedure often defended as an effective means to achieve pain relief, certainly may not be as benign a procedure as often suggested, and this is a factor worth considering in the planning of joint capsulotomies.

One of the most notable, yet poorly recognized, advantages of arthroscopy is the ability to observe, manipulate, and correct problems within the joint without creating substantial damage to capsular innervation. This probably explains why procedures done arthroscopically tend to recover function faster than those performed through an open approach. If a condition can be solved arthroscopically, open surgery is certainly not indicated. There are instances, however, where an open approach is mandatory. Depending on the location of the anatomic structure to be addressed, one may choose from various surgical approaches.

INNERVATION OF THE DISTAL RADIOULNAR JOINT

According to Gupta and colleagues[8] and Shigemitsu and colleagues,[9] the palmar capsule, anterior radioulnar, and ulnolunate ligaments are mostly innervated by branches of the ulnar nerve. Branches from the anterior interosseous nerve (AIN) are additionally found to innervate the volar DRUJ capsule,[10,11] but detailed microscopic studies have not disclosed AIN contributions to

[a] Institut Kaplan, Passeig de la Bonanova, 9, 2on 2ª, 08022 Barcelona, Spain
[b] Hand & Foot Reconstructive Surgery Center, Karolinska Institutet, Storangsv. 10, 115 42 Stockholm, Sweden
* Corresponding author.
E-mail address: garciaelias@institut-kaplan.com

Hand Clin 26 (2010) 477–483
doi:10.1016/j.hcl.2010.05.001
0749-0712/10/$ – see front matter © 2010 Elsevier Inc. All rights reserved.

the actual DRUJ ligaments.[8] The dorsal DRUJ capsule, the posterior radioulnar ligament, and the dorsal ulnocarpal capsule are innervated by branches of the posterior interosseous nerve. Everything else, including the meniscus homolog, the foveal attachment of the TFC, the prestyloid recess, and the ulnotriquetral ligament is innervated by articular extensions of the dorsal sensory branches of the ulnar nerve.[8,9] The central portion of the TFC, the so-called discus articularis, is avascular and aneural, explaining why central TFC perforations may remain asymptomatic unless they are associated with another local injury causing synovitis.

When discussing surgical approaches to the TFC, certain aspects of the DRUJ innervation are important to note. First, most ulnar branches of the posterior interosseous nerve enter the joint along the dorsal margin of the TFC. Consequently this structure will be denervated if the TFC is detached off the dorsal capsule. Second, no matter how the DRUJ is surgically approached, it is always essential to identify and carefully protect the articular extensions of the dorsal branch of the ulnar nerve. These branches are the only ones that transmit proprioceptive information from the most important functional portions of the TFC.[9] Finally, there is a safe zone through which the joint can be entered without creating substantial denervation; namely, the zone between the meniscus homolog and the ulnotriquetral ligament, and proximally along the ulnar insertion of the palmar radioulnar capsule.

With this information in mind, several surgical alternatives have been investigated in cadaver specimens at the Anatomy Department of the University of Barcelona, Spain. This article describes 3 surgical approaches to the DRUJ—dorsoulnar, ulnar, and palmar—with emphasis on their respective ability to expose different DRUJ structures, and their morbidity in terms of sensory innervation of the joint.

DORSOULNAR APPROACH

Most surgical approaches to the DRUJ described in the literature are dorsal or dorsoulnar.[12–15] Bower's approach involves 2 retinacular flaps, 1 radially based and 1 ulnarly based. The medial edge of the radially based flap overlies the thin ECU sheath, an important structure that may be inadvertently damaged with rising of this retinacular flap. The capsular incision is C-shaped, creating an ulnar-based capsular flap with a distal incision along the proximal edge of the dorsal radioulnar ligament; therefore, the distal aspect of the TFC is not well visualized.[12] The technique of Berger and Bishop[13] involves an inverted-V capsulotomy based on the line of the dorsal radiotriquetral ligament and the edge of the VI compartment. This approach only visualizes the distal aspect of the TFC and lunotriquetral joint and does not allow access to the proximal aspect of the TFC or DRUJ, because any proximal extension of the vertical limb of the capsular incision would disrupt the ECU sheath. Tubiana and colleagues[14] recommends division of the ECU sheath to expose the underlying capsule. It is the authors' belief, however, that the ECU and its surrounding stabilizing structures should not be violated during the surgical approach.[6] Webhe's approach[15] to the ulnar side of the wrist is similar to what is described here, except that the TFC is not dissected off the capsule, thus limiting the overall exposure of the DRUJ joint including the TFC.

The dorsoulnar approach suggested provides excellent exposure to the ulnocarpal and radioulnar joints, the dorsal edge of the TFC, the meniscus homolog, and the dorsal aspect of the lunotriquetral joint.[16] The major drawback of this approach is that it denervates the dorsal capsule almost completely and denervates the posterior radioulnar ligament partly. If carefully executed, the dorsal branches of the posterior interosseous nerve supplying the ulnar head and the area adjacent to the foveal attachment of the TFC may be preserved.

The dorsoulnar approach described was first published by the first author of this article in 2003,[16] and it is mostly indicated in chronic DRUJ dysfunctions with joint degeneration requiring some sort of salvage procedure. In such instances, proprioception stabilization of the joint has long been altered, and denervation may even be beneficial for its pain-controlling effects. This approach is also indicated when surgery is planned to solve pathology to the ECU tendon sheath. What follows is a step-by-step description of this approach.

> Step 1: A 2-cm oblique incision at the level of the distal corner of the ulnar head is used to identify and protect the dorsal branch of the ulnar nerve (DBU) (**Fig. 1**A). This incision is prolonged proximally and distally, in a zigzag fashion. Using a blunt dissection, the subcutaneous tissue is elevated en bloc and all small perforating vessels are coagulated. Anomalous transverse branches toward the radius proximal to the ulnar styloid are not uncommon, and need to be identified and protected.[6]

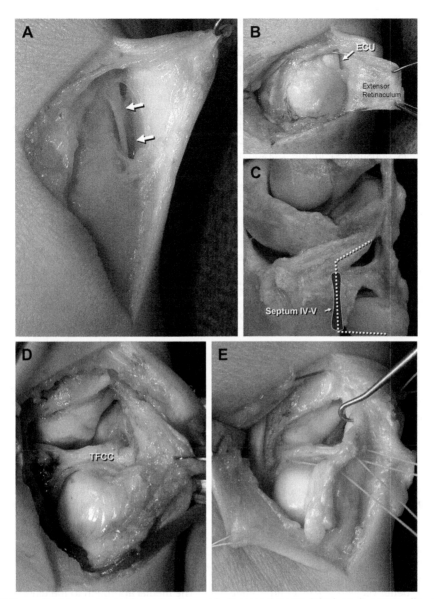

Fig. 1. (*A–E*) Dorsoulnar approach to the radioulnar and ulnocarpal joints. (*A*) Blunt dissection allows identification and protection of the DBU (*arrows*). (*B*) An ulnar-based extensor retinaculum flap is elevated uncovering the subretinacular extracapsular space. The ECU tendon is maintained in the dorsal groove of the ulna by the ECU subsheath, forming the VI extensor compartment. (*C*) Schematic representation in the cadaver of the ulnar-based capsulotomy, with a vertical incision along the septum between the IV and V extensor compartment, a distal incision along the fibers of the dorsal radiotriquetral ligament, and a proximal incision aiming at the neck of the ulna. (*D*) The capsular flap is elevated by sectioning its inner connections with the dorsal edge of the TFC complex (TFCC). Further excision of the synovial tissue that occupies the dorsoulnar space of the ulnocarpal joint allows excellent visualization of this joint. (*E*) When closing the capsular flap, it is important to reestablish the capsular connection with the TFC by means of sutures. This enhances the so-called trampoline effect of the TFC, providing further DRUJ stability.

Step 2: The fifth extensor compartment is released following its oblique course. The septum between the fourth and fifth compartments is sectioned at its most superficial level, leaving some soft tissue attached to the radius for later repair. The fourth compartment artery, which often lies within this septum, needs to be identified and protected, or coagulated if damage is unavoidable.

Step 3: Once released, the extensor digiti quinti (EDQ) is retracted radially and the floor of the fifth compartment is carefully incised to enter the extracapsular subretinacular space. Proximal and distal transverse incisions along the fibers of the extensor retinaculum are then made to create an ulnarly based retinacular flap, which is carefully elevated to uncover the ECU tendon. In normal wrists, the ECU tendon is constrained in the dorsoulnar groove of the ulna by a thin layer of collagen tissue, the so-called ECU subsheath, which is independent from the extensor retinaculum (**Fig. 1**B).

Step 4: Using the dorsal prominence of the triquetrum as an anatomic landmark, and starting at the distal edge of the previously incised IV-V septum, an oblique incision is created following the direction of the dorsal radiotriquetral ligament, similar to the "fiber-splitting technique" to explore the proximal carpal row (**Fig. 1**C).[13] This incision is prolonged proximally along the septum to the level of the radial metaphysis where it angles ulnarly aiming at the proximal corner of the radioulnar capsule. This capsular flap is elevated by sectioning its dorsal connection to the TFC. By doing so, this portion of TFC becomes denervated. The lateral insertion of the capsule onto the radial edge of the ECU groove need not be detached unless the tendon has some pathology that needs to be specifically explored. Indeed, exploring the ECU from outside, by incising the ECU subsheath, is not recommended because it may result in scar retraction and stenosing tenosynovitis, or in healing insufficiency and ECU subluxation.

Step 5: To better visualize the ulnocarpal joint, the triangular distal expansion of the TFC complex, the so-called ulnomeniscal homolog,[17] can be excised (**Fig. 1**D). This structure is formed by highly vascularized loose connective tissue in which excision needs to be followed by careful coagulation of any bleeding vessel. The stabilizing importance of this "meniscoid" is minimal, because its excision is recommended if there is a need for maximizing exposure of the ulnocarpal space.

Step 6: To preserve as much of the normal anatomy as possible, it is important to reconstruct the different layers as if they were independent structures. The dorsal edge of the TFC is sutured to the capsular flap with the knots secured outside of the capsule (**Fig. 1**E). The dorsal radiotriquetral ligament is sutured in a side-to-side fashion. The remnant of the IV-V septum is used to close the lateral portion of the capsular incision. The ECU subsheath remains intact and in its groove on the dorsum of the distal ulna. The extensor retinaculum is repaired over the EDQ tendon. The septum between the fifth compartment and the extracapsular infraretinaculum space is not reconstructed.

ULNAR APPROACH

Approaching the wrist through its medial border is seldom recommended because it provides very limited exposure to the joint while implying substantial risk of damaging the articular extensions of the DBU. These branches emerge at the level of the ulnar styloid and have a transverse course across the extensor retinaculum, perforating the dorsomedial capsule between the ECU and the ulnar styloid, toward the medial corner of the TFC. Between the 2 insertions of the TFC (foveal and ulnar styloid insertions), there is a well-vascularized zone where these branches divide, forming a network of dendrites innervating the most important sectors of the TFC complex.[9] Aside from the risk of denervating the TFC, and eventually creating painful neuromas there, this approach does not offer good exposure to the ulnocarpal joint because of the presence of the ulnar styloid, which covers the medial corner of the joint, and the ECU tendon, which occupies its dorsoulnar corner. Mobilizing the tendon to facilitate better exposure to the joint is certainly not recommended because this would imply releasing the ECU subsheath that maintains this tendon stable relative to the ulna.

The medial approach to the ulnocarpal space is used only in 6 particular situations: (1) as an entry point for irrigation of the joint during wrist arthroscopy, (2) to secure sutures outside the joint in some arthroscopically guided TFC reconstructions, (3) to excise the meniscus homolog should this become fibrotic and impinge the triquetrum, (4) to release pressure on the medial border of the carpus by an excessively taut extensor retinaculum, the so-called TILT syndrome,[18] (5) to excise the tip of the ulnar styloid when abnormally prominent, and (6) to treat dysesthesia secondary to injury of the DBU.

When indicated, the ulnar approach is used as follows. A small medial transverse or zigzag incision between the ulnar corner of the pisiform and the dorsoulnar prominence of the ECU tendon is made. Careful blunt dissection of the subcutaneous tissue allows exposure of the DBU. Care is taken to localize and protect the 2 or 3 small branches that arise from the nerve at this level to penetrate the transverse fibers of the extensor retinaculum. Once these structures are protected, the extensor retinaculum is divided vertically, leaving the perforating nerves in the dorsal portion of retinaculum. From that point, the ulnocarpal joint may be approached in 3 ways: distal to the ulnar styloid, around the palmar edge to the ulnar styloid, or between the ECU and the ulnar styloid. The last option is not recommended, as the risk of damaging the perforating articular branches is too high. The first option is preferred if the goal of the procedure is to trim the tip of the ulnar styloid. Once the limited styloidectomy is done, the meniscus homolog may be excised without endangering the DRUJ stability; this allows good exposure of the medial corner of the triquetrum.[18] Approaching the joint around the palmar corner of the ulnar styloid is recommended when there is a need for an early synovectomy in rheumatoid disease; just palmar to the ulnar styloid there is the prestyloid recess, a synovial fluid–filled articular extension where the destructive process often starts.

PALMAR APPROACH

Despite the recent advances concerning the understanding of the functional importance of the palmar radio-ulno-carpal capsule and ligaments,[5,19] little attention has been paid to developing volar approaches to explore and/or repair these structures. The first description of a volar approach to the radioulnar joint was published in 1998 by Kleinman and Graham[20] to treat posttraumatic limitations of supination. Kleinman and Graham suggested a volar "silhouette" resection of the DRUJ capsule to eliminate pathologic thickened tissue that prevents normal forearm rotation. Moritomo[21] also recommended a volar approach in cases with foveal tears of the TFC, with normal styloid insertion. In that case, the injury is approached by means of a transverse capsulotomy of the DRUJ plus an opening of the ulnocarpal joint between the ulnar styloid and the ulnotriquetral ligament. In the authors' opinion, a carefully executed volar approach not only provides excellent exposure to the joint but also, and most importantly, is the soundest approach from the viewpoint of sensory preservation of the joint. Indeed, as already mentioned, there is a safe zone between the ulnar styloid and the ulnotriquetral ligament, free of sensory nerves, through which the joint can be entered without creating substantial denervation. What follows is a step-by-step description of the volar surgical approach to the DRUJ that the authors have developed in the cadaver laboratory and that is being currently used in their practices in most DRUJ conditions requiring open surgery.

Step 1: A zigzag incision across the 2 skin creases, located ulnar to the insertion of the flexor carpi ulnaris (FCU) onto the pisiform, is used to identify and protect the DBU (**Fig. 2**A). If required, this incision may be prolonged distally following the medial contour of the pisiform and the abductor digiti minimi muscle, and proximally by means of a longitudinal incision parallel to the FCU.

Step 2: Gentle retraction of the DBU allows exposure of the superficial fascia, which distally blends with thick transverse fibers coming from the dorsum as palmar extensions of the extensor retinaculum inserting onto the medial aspect of the pisiform. A longitudinal incision of this superficial fascia allows entry to the subretinacular space, filled with fat tissue, adjacent to pisotriquetral joint distally, and covering the DRUJ capsule proximally (**Fig. 2**B).

Step 3: At this point, it is mandatory to use blunt dissection to identify and protect the main trunk of the ulnar nerve, which lies deep to the FCU tendon. Once this nerve and its dorsal branch have been protected, the deep fascia that covers the PQ muscle can be exposed. Distal to this muscle lies the volar surface of the radioulnar and ulnocarpal capsule. Lateral to the muscle, the ulnar border of the pisotriquetral joint may be observed and easily mobilized, particularly with wrist flexion. The location of the interval between the radioulnar and ulnocarpal joint spaces can be easily recognized by further supinating the forearm: the convex ulnar head will be more prominent as it slides palmarly relative to the sigmoid notch. Its distal edge indicates the location of the anterior border of the TFC.

Step 4: To obtain further exposure of the ulnocarpal space, it is helpful to incise the medial capsule of the pisotriquetral joint and supinate the pisiform relative to the triquetrum (**Fig. 2**C). By rotating the pisiform about its distal ligament connections, not only can the pisotriquetral joint surfaces be explored but also the ulnar edge of the ulnotriquetral ligament can be made

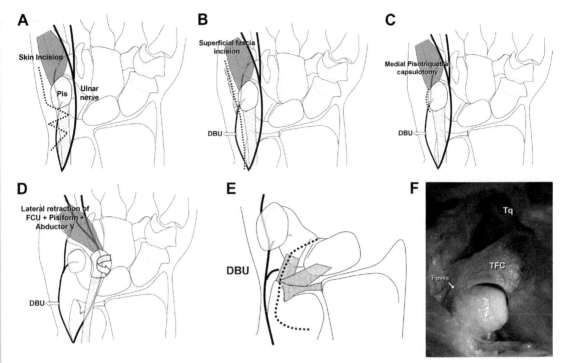

Fig. 2. (*A–F*) Palmar approach to the TFC. (*A*) Zigzag skin incision proximal to the pisiform bone (Pis). (*B*) Recognition and protection of the DBU. Longitudinal incision of the superficial fascia, including the medial and palmar extension of the extensor retinaculum. (*C*) To facilitate further exposure, the medial capsule of the pisotriquetral joint may be opened. (*D*) This exposure allows a supination subluxation of the pisiform and a better exposure of the ulnocarpal capsule. (*E*) Radial-based capsulotomy with a distal incision along the fibers of the ulnotriquetral ligament, a vertical incision along the ulnar attachment of the capsule, and a proximal transverse incision aiming at the proximal border of the sigmoid notch. (*F*) This capsulotomy allows wide exposure of the palmar aspect of the TFC, including its relationship with the triquetrum (Tq) and its insertion onto the fovea.

evident (**Fig. 2**D). Indeed, often there is an anatomic communication of the pisitriquetral to the ulnocarpal joint space located between the ulnotriquetral ligament and the meniscus homolog. This communication will be the landmark used to design the ulnocarpal capsulotomy.

Step 5: As mentioned, most of the palmar DRUJ capsule and anterior radioulnar ligament is innervated by branches arising from the ulnar nerve, with additional capsular contributions from the AIN. Any capsular incision along the radial border of the sigmoid notch will necessarily denervate these structures. To preserve the sensory innervation, and knowing that there is a safe zone, free of sensory nerves, along the medial insertion of the DRUJ capsule and ulnar to the ulnotriquetral ligament, 2 radially based capsular flaps have been developed; one offering the widest possible view of the TFC insertion, another exposing only the ulnar head.

Radio-Ulno-Carpal Capsulotomy

This extended capsulotomy is defined by 3 incisions: (1) a proximal transverse incision, distal to the PQ, (2) a longitudinal incision along the ulnar insertion of the DRUJ capsule, following the medial border of the protruding ulnar head, extended distally up to the level where the ulnar head prominence disappears, and (3) an oblique incision from the distal end of the previous incision to the proximal border of the pisotriquetral joint (**Fig. 2**E). The last incision would be a fiber-splitting type of incision, as it is intended to follow the direction of most ulnar fibers of the ulnotriquetral ligament. The capsular flap is elevated by incising its inner connections to the anterior fibers of the ulnotriquetral ligament and to the palmar edge of the TFC, which in this location consists of the palmar radioulnar ligament (**Fig. 2**F). It is obvious that the deeper this connection is severed, the thicker will be the portion of ulnotriquetral ligament detached. Despite this being a wide ligament, caution is recommended and the exposure should be limited strictly to the necessary.

Radioulnar Capsulotomy

When there is no need to expose the ulnocarpal space but only the radioulnar articulation, a less-extended radially based capsulotomy is preferred. In this case, the proximal and medial capsular incisions are identical as with the more-extended capsulotomy described. The distal incision in this case is transverse along the distal border of the ulnar head, creating a capsular window that is elevated to uncover only the ulnar head, should this be the only structure that needs to be addressed.

SUMMARY

In addition to their important stabilizing function, DRUJ ligaments also have a proprioceptive function in controlling the dynamic neuromuscular stability of the DRUJ. By careful planning and meticulous execution of surgical incisions to approach the DRUJ, the nerve endings innervating the capsule and DRUJ ligaments may be safeguarded, thus preserving the proprioceptive function of the joint.

REFERENCES

1. Lephart SM, Riemann BL, Fu FH. Introduction to the sensorimotor system. In: Lephart SM, Fu FH, editors. Proprioception and neuromuscular control in joint stability. Champaign (IL): Human Kinetics; 2000. p. xvii–xxiv.
2. Riemann BL, Lephart SM. The Sensorimotor system, part i: the physiologic basis of functional joint stability. J Athl Train 2002;37(1):71–9.
3. Hagert E, Garcia-Elias M, Forsgren S, et al. Immunohistochemical analysis of wrist ligament innervation in relation to their structural composition. J Hand Surg Am 2007;32(1):30–6.
4. Hagert E, Persson JK, Werner M, et al. Evidence of wrist proprioceptive reflexes elicited after stimulation of the scapholunate interosseous ligament. J Hand Surg Am 2009;34(4):642–51.
5. Garcia-Elias M. Soft-tissue anatomy and relationships about the distal ulna. Hand Clin 1998;14(2):165–76.
6. Garcia-Elias M. Management of soft tissue contractures around the distal radioulnar joint. In: Slutsky DJ, editor. Principles and practice of wrist surgery. Philadelphia: Elsevier; 2009. p. 327–34.
7. Gordon KD, Pardo RD, Johnson JA, et al. Electromyographic activity and strength during maximum isometric pronation and supination efforts in healthy adults. J Orthop Res 2004;22(1):208–13.
8. Gupta R, Nelson SD, Baker J, et al. The innervation of the triangular fibrocartilage complex: nitric acid maceration rediscovered. Plast Reconstr Surg 2001;107(1):135–9.
9. Shigemitsu T, Tobe M, Mizutani K, et al. Innervation of the triangular fibrocartilage complex of the human wrist: quantitative immunohistochemical study. Anat Sci Int 2007;82(3):127–32.
10. Ferreres A, Suso S, Ordi J, et al. Wrist denervation. Anatomical considerations. J Hand Surg Br 1995; 20(6):761–8.
11. Fukumoto K, Kojima T, Kinoshita Y, et al. An anatomic study of the innervation of the wrist joint and Wilhelm's technique for denervation. J Hand Surg Am 1993;18(3):484–9.
12. Bowers MW. The distal radioulnar joint. In: Green DP, Hotchkiss RN, Pedersen WC, editors. Green's operative hand surgery. Philadelphia: Churchill Livingstone; 1999. p. 986–1032.
13. Berger RA, Bishop AT. A fiber-splitting capsulotomy technique for dorsal exposure of the wrist. Tech Hand Up Extrem Surg 1997;1(1):2–10.
14. Tubiana R, McCullough CJ, Masquelet AC. Wrist: extensor aspect and carpus. In: Tubiana R, McCullough CJ, Masquelet AC, editors. An atlas of surgical exposures of the upper extremity. London: Martin Dunitz; 1990. p. 230–2.
15. Webhe MA. Surgical approach to the ulnar wrist. J Hand Surg Am 1986;11(4):509–12.
16. Garcia-Elias M, Smith DE, Llusa M. Surgical approach to the triangular fibrocartilage complex. Tech Hand Up Extrem Surg 2003;7(4):134–40.
17. Buck FM, Gheno R, Nico MA, et al. Ulnomeniscal homologue of the wrist: correlation of anatomic and MR imaging findings. Radiology 2009;253(3): 771–9.
18. Watson HK, Weinzweig J. Triquetral impingement ligament tear (TILT). J Hand Surg Br 1999;24(3): 321–4.
19. Kleinman WB. Stability of the distal radioulnar joint: biomechanics, pathophysiology, physical diagnosis, and restoration of function what we have learned in 25 years. J Hand Surg Am 2007; 32(7):1086–106.
20. Kleinman WB, Graham TJ. The distal radioulnar joint capsule: clinical anatomy and role in posttraumatic limitation of forearm rotation. J Hand Surg Am 1998;23(4):588–99.
21. Moritomo H. Advantages of open repair of a foveal tear of the triangular fibrocartilage complex via a palmar surgical approach. Tech Hand Up Extrem Surg 2009;13(4):176–81.

Arthroscopic and Open Repair of the TFCC

Rudy Kovachevich, MD, Bassem T. Elhassan, MD*

KEYWORDS

- Triangular fibrocartilage complex • TFCC
- Arthroscopic repair • Open repair

The triangular fibrocartilage complex (TFCC) is an important stabilizer of the distal radioulnar joint (DRUJ) and load absorber between the distal ulna and the volar carpus. The complex was first described by Palmer and Werner[1] as a group of functionally related, but anatomically distinct soft-tissue structures in the ulnar side of the wrist. The TFCC consists of the triangular fibrocartilage proper (the articular disk), palmar and dorsal radioulnar ligaments, meniscal homolog, the ulnar collateral ligament, and the extensor carpi ulnaris (ECU) tendon subsheath. The anatomic complexity of this area places it at substantial risk for injury and degeneration. Injury to the TFCC can result in vague ulnar-sided wrist pain, which may be associated with a palpable click with forearm rotation.

The most problematic condition arising from soft-tissue injury of this important structure is DRUJ instability. This joint, a diarthroidal trochoid articulation, provides a distal link between the radius and ulna. An incongruent articulation, only approximately 20% of its stability is produced by osseous articular contact,[2] this resulting from the curvature of the sigmoid notch of the radius being larger than that of the radial border of the ulna. Soft-tissue structures of the TFCC, in turn, play a critical role in intrinsic joint stability. The DRUJ is primarily stabilized by the dorsal and palmar radioulnar ligaments, which originate from the fovea of the ulna (**Fig. 1**). The palmar radioulnar ligament is the major constraint to palmar translation and supination of the distal radius relative to the ulna.

Dorsal translation and pronation, in turn, is primarily constrained by the dorsal radioulnar ligament.[2,3] The distal portion of the interosseous membrane, extensor retinaculum, and the muscle-tendon units that cross the longitudinal axis of rotation of the forearm have also been shown to provide supplemental stability.[4]

The blood supply to the TFCC originates from the terminal portions of the anterior and posterior interosseous arteries of the forearm. Similar to the human knee meniscus, the vascularity of the articular disk has significant anatomic variability that has direct implications for treatment and tissue-healing potential. The peripheral palmar, ulnar, and dorsal components are well vascularized with good healing potential with direct repair, whereas the central and radial components are poorly vascularized and often require debridement.[5,6]

The treatment of these injuries consists initially of standard nonsurgical measures including activity modification, temporary splint or cast immobilization of the wrist and forearm, nonsteroidal anti-inflammatory medication, corticosteroid joint injections, and occupational therapy modalities. When conservative treatment has been exhausted, or in specific situations of acute DRUJ instability or unstable and displaced fractures, operative treatment may be considered. Operative management includes open or arthroscopic debridement, repair and/or, in TFCC injuries associated with degenerative changes, ulnar unloading procedures.[7–9]

Department of Orthopedic Surgery, Mayo Clinic, 200 First Street Southwest, Rochester, MN 55905, USA
* Corresponding author.
E-mail address: elhassan.bassem@mayo.edu

Hand Clin 26 (2010) 485–494
doi:10.1016/j.hcl.2010.07.003
0749-0712/10/$ — see front matter © 2010 Published by Elsevier Inc.

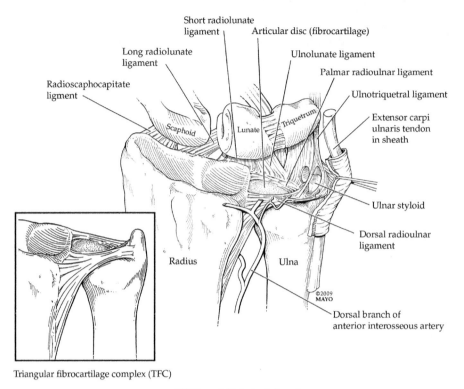

Triangular fibrocartilage complex (TFC)

TFC and Related Anatomy

Fig. 1. Details of the triangular fibrocartilage complex (TFCC) and related anatomy. (*From* Carlsen B, Rizzo M, Moran S. Soft-tissue injuries associated with distal radius fractures. Operat Tech Orthop 2009;19(2):109; with permission.)

This article reviews the diagnosis, classification, and treatment options (including open and arthroscopic techniques) of TFCC injuries.

DIAGNOSIS
Examination

TFCC tears are the most common source of ulnar-sided wrist pain. To accurately diagnose TFCC injury from other ulnar-sided cause of wrist pain, one must start with a complete history, perform a detailed clinical examination, and accurately interpret appropriate diagnostic tests. The clinical presentation of a patient with a TFCC tear primarily produces ulnar-sided mechanical wrist pain worsened by motions and activities that reproduce the mechanism of injury or load the ulnar side of the wrist. Patients with an anatomic basis for ulnar-sided wrist pain typically localize this pain to the ulnar side of the wrist. The most common mechanism of injury to the TFCC occurs with axial loading, ulnar deviation, and forced extremes of forearm rotation. Injury may also be associated with localized swelling, crepitus, grip weakness, or a sense of instability.

Physical examination begins with inspection of the involved extremity. The examination should be performed with the patient on the opposite side of a hand table with the elbow resting on the table and the fingers pointing toward the ceiling. All observations or findings should be compared with the opposite side because some findings may be symmetric. The wrist, forearm, and elbow should be examined for previous surgical scars. Prominence of the ulna in a volar or dorsal direction may indicate instability of the DRUJ.

Palpation of the wrist should then be performed in a systematic fashion to isolate anatomic structures that could be causing the patient's symptoms. Tenderness over any specific anatomic structure suggests a possible origin. The TFCC is best palpated in the soft spot between the ulnar styloid, flexor carpi ulnaris tendon, volar surface of the ulnar head, and pisiform (**Fig. 2**). This area has been described as the fovea by Tay and colleagues,[10] and exquisite tenderness with deep palpation of this area that replicates the patient's complaint of pain in character and location compared with the contralateral side is considered a positive "ulna fovea sign." This examination

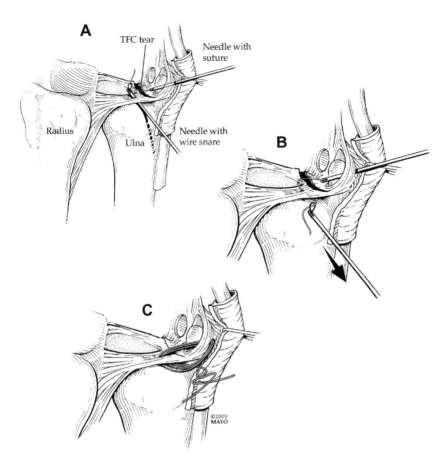

Arthroscopic Repair

Fig. 2. (*A*) The TFCC origin is best palpated in the soft spot between the ulnar styloid process, flexor carpi ulnaris tendon, volar surface of the ulnar head (covered by the examiner index finger tip), and pisiform. (*B*) The examining thumb tip is pressed distally and deep into the soft spot between the ulnar styloid process, flexor carpi ulnaris, volar surface of the ulnar head, and the pisiform. Exquisite tenderness on palpation compared with the contralateral side may indicate either foveal detachment of the TFCC or ulnotriquetral ligament split tear (*C*). (*From* Tay SC, Tomita K, Berger RA. The "Ulnar fovea sign" for defining ulnar wrist pain: an analysis of sensitivity and specificity. J Hand Surg Am 2007;32(4):438–44; with permission.)

finding was critically analyzed in a cohort of 272 patients, and was found to have a sensitivity of 95.2% and specificity of 86.5% for either ulnotriquetral ligament tears or TFCC foveal disruptions at the time of wrist arthroscopy. Other provocative maneuvers that can produce pain within the TFCC include ulnocarpal stress testing, hypersupination, and DRUJ loading.

The stability of the DRUJ also needs to be tested. Stress testing is performed by stabilizing the ulna with one hand and translating the radius in volar and dorsal directions. This maneuver should be performed in neutral, pronation, and supination forearm positions, and the amplitude and end point firmness should be noted and compared with the contralateral extremity.

Finally, selective local anesthetic and/or corticosteroid injections can be important adjuncts to confirming pathologic changes found on physical examination. Suspected TFCC injuries should respond to intra-articular injection to the ulnocarpal joint.

Imaging Studies

Numerous imaging modalities are available for the evaluation of TFCC injuries, and appropriate studies can assist in establishing a diagnosis and treatment plan. Plain radiographs should initially be performed as part of a complete wrist trauma evaluation. Radiographs should include neutral rotation posteroanterior, neutral rotation lateral, and oblique views. These views are useful as screening tools to look for evidence of fracture, carpal alignment or instability, arthritis, ulnar variance, and DRUJ instability, which could point toward other causes of ulnar-sided wrist pain.

The gold standard advanced imaging modality traditionally used to assess TFCC disruption was triple injection arthrography. However, numerous studies evaluating findings on arthrography compared with findings during wrist arthroscopy have shown decreased accuracy and relatively high false-negative rates[11,12] as well as poor correlation of arthrographic findings with clinical symptoms.[13–15] Chung and colleagues,[12] in their study comparing wrist arthrography with arthroscopy in 150 patients, found agreement between the 2 methods in only 42%, a change in arthrographic diagnosis after arthroscopy in 58%, and an 80% false-negative rate in those with normal arthrographic findings after arthroscopy.

In recent years, arthrography has been largely supplanted by magnetic resonance imaging (MRI) as the advanced imaging modality of choice for the evaluation of TFCC injuries (**Fig. 3**). Optimal MRI of the wrist is performed with use of a dedicated wrist coil and a high-field strength magnet.[16] 1.5-T magnets have been routinely used in the majority of recent studies; however, new 3.0-T magnets have emerged and preliminary studies have shown increased diagnostic accuracy.[17,18] Early studies demonstrated MRI having poor accuracy rates for localization of TFCC tears.[19,20] Potter and colleagues[21] showed in a more recent study using a dedicated surface coil and high-resolution 3-dimensional gradient techniques a 97% accuracy of MRI in detection and 92% localization capability for TFCC tears. The efficacy of MRI to detect and localize TFCC injuries is also highly dependent on the experience of those interpreting these MRI studies.[22]

Although imaging modalities such as MRI and arthrography are helpful in the diagnosis of TFCC tears, the gold standard modality is direct intra-articular visualization by wrist arthroscopy. The use of wrist arthroscopy for evaluation of disorders involving the TFCC is one of its most common uses.[23–25] Arthroscopic evaluation allows characterization of TFCC tears and immediate treatment as indicated.

Classification

TFCC tears were classified by Palmer as traumatic (Type 1) and degenerative (Type 2), outlined in **Table 1**.[26] Each group was subsequently divided into subtypes, with lesions classified as Type 1 based on the anatomic location of tissue disruption and Type 2 based on the extent of the degenerative process.

Type 1A lesions consist of central tears within the substance of the fibrocartilage disk, and are the most common type of traumatic tear (**Fig. 4**). These lesions are not generally associated with instability or altered kinematics of the DRUJ,[27,28] and typically involve a sagittal tear in the radial portion of the disk; however, more complex tears can involve the entire disk.

Type 1B lesions consist of peripheral tears of the TFCC from its insertion into the distal ulna (see **Fig. 4**). These injuries may be ligamentous avulsion injuries from the fovea or bony through the ulnar styloid. Instability of the DRUJ is common and must be carefully evaluated.

Type 1C lesions are rare, high-energy injuries that involve the volar ulnar extrinsic ligament complex, which consists of the ulnolunate, ulnotriquetral, and/or ulnocapitate ligaments. The robust nature of these ligaments makes them resistant to injury and it takes a substantial force to cause a disruption, such as a radiocarpal dislocation. Because of this, these lesions are commonly associated with DRUJ instability. Ligamentous

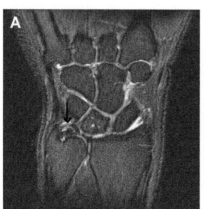
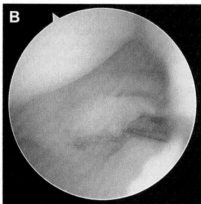

Fig. 3. (*A*) MRI scan showing central of the TFCC (*arrow*). (*B*) Arthroscopic picture of the patient in **Fig. 3**A, demonstrating the central tear of TFCC.

Table 1 Palmer classification of TFCC tears	
Type of Tear	**Description**
Type 1: Acute Traumatic	
1A	Isolated central TFCC articular disk perforation
1B	Peripheral ulnar-sided TFCC tear (with or without ulnar styloid fracture)
1C	Distal TFCC disruption (disruption from distal ulnocarpal ligaments)
1D	Radial TFCC disruption (with or without sigmoid notch fracture)
Type 2: Degenerative	
2A	TFCC wear
2B	TFCC wear with lunate and/or ulnar chondromalacia
2C	TFCC perforation with lunate and/or ulnar chondromalacia
2D	TFCC perforation with lunate and/or ulnar chondromalacia and with lunotriquetral ligament perforation
2E	TFCC perforation with lunate and/or ulnar chondromalacia, lunotriquetral ligament perforation and ulnocarpal arthritis

radioulnar ligaments. These uncommon injuries are at high risk for DRUJ instability.

Degenerative, or Type 2 tears, are a result of chronic loading of the ulnar aspect of the wrist and ulnar impaction syndrome. Pathologic changes within this classification worsen progressively, as can be seen in **Table 1**. These changes begin with TFCC thinning and wear, with progression to chondromalacia of the ulnar lunate and ulnar head. Perforations within the TFCC and then the ulnotriquetral ligament develop and finally progress to ulnocarpal arthritis. Palmer's classification scheme implies that each type of tear occurs in isolation; however, clinical studies have shown that multiple areas of the TFCC may tear in a single injury.[29]

Treatment

The treatment of TFCC injuries consists initially of nonsurgical measures including activity modification, temporary splint or cast immobilization of the wrist and forearm, nonsteroidal anti-inflammatory medication, corticosteroid joint injections, and occupational therapy. When conservative treatment has been exhausted, or in specific situations of acute DRUJ instability or unstable and displaced fractures, operative treatment may be considered. Arthroscopic and open techniques for TFCC debridement or repair have been described for the treatment of acute and degenerative tears. The decision for properly treating these lesions is usually made based on the location and size of the tear.

disruption can also be associated with marginal fractures of the radius, which also often results in DRUJ instability.

Type 1D lesions are TFCC radial-sided detachments from the sigmoid notch of the radius. These lesions occur only through bone, and are typically associated with marginal sigmoid notch fractures and the insertion sites of the dorsal and palmar

Arthroscopic Debridement

Palmer Type 1A tears that fail conservative measures are the lesions most amenable to

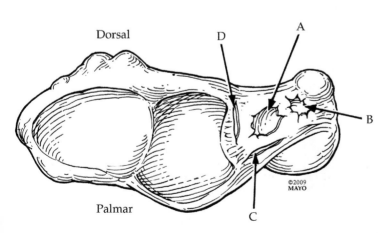

Common TFC Tears

Fig. 4. Palmar classification of traumatic TFCC tear. (*A*) Central tear. (*B*) Peripheral tear of the TFCC from its insertion into the distal ulnar. (*C*) Tear of the volar ulnar extrinsic ligament complex. (*D*) Radial detachment of the TFCC from the sigmoid notch of the radius. (*From* Carlsen B, Rizzo M, Moran S. Soft-tissue injuries associated with distal radius fractures. Operat Tech Orthop 2009;19 (2):107–18; with permission.)

arthroscopic debridement. Tears within the central disk typically create an unstable flap of tissue that can catch on surfaces within the joint. The goal of debridement is to remove all loose flap components and create a stable rim of TFCC when stressed with a probe (**Fig. 5**). Biomechanical studies have shown that up to 80% of the disk substance can be resected without creating iatrogenic instability.[2,30]

Visualization of the TFCC is performed through a standard wrist arthroscopy technique using the dorsal 3-4 portal. Probe examination of the articular disk with the so-called trampoline test allows the surgeon to assess the tension and rebound ability of the disk. Laxity and absence of disk rebound indicates detachment at one or more anatomic insertion sites. Foveal insertional fiber integrity of the radioulnar ligaments can also be assessed through this portal to rule out an associated peripheral (Type 1B) tear. Debridement is then performed through the 6R portal and may be performed with various arthroscopic instruments including 2.0-mm or 3.0-mm motorized shavers, radiofrequency ablation probes, ultrasonic/laser devices, or arthroscopic knives/punches. No comparative studies have been performed for these specific debridement devices.

The success rates of arthroscopic debridement of Type 1A TFCC tears have ranged from 66% to 87%.[9,31–34] Arthroscopic debridement of ulnar-positive wrists has met with less successful results. Failure rates of 13% to 60% have been documented in the literature.[9,33,35] Higher failures have been postulated to be secondary to an underlying degenerative TFCC on top of the acute Type 1A tear. Treatment in this scenario would involve arthroscopic debridement of the unstable flap tear in conjunction with an ulnocarpal unloading procedure, as is discussed below. Hulsizer and colleagues[36] evaluated 97 patients with central or nondetached ulnar peripheral tears of the TFCC and performed arthroscopic debridement. Of these 97, 13 had persistent pain in the TFCC region for more than 3 months after surgery. The investigators performed 2-mm ulnar-shortening osteotomies on these treatment failure patients, regardless of the wrist ulnar variance, and increased their overall success rate from 87% to 99%. The determination of mild, symptomatic degenerative changes associated with Type 1A tears may affect outcomes of arthroscopic debridement in all patients.

Arthroscopic Repair

Ulnar-sided peripheral tears within the vascular zone of the TFCC are most amenable to arthroscopic or open repair. These types of tears are most characteristic of Palmer 1B lesions. Numerous arthroscopic techniques have been described; including inside-out, outside-in, and all-inside techniques.[37–39] To date, there have been no direct-comparison studies between techniques; however, all have been found to be effective with good results.[40]

Arthroscopic repair is performed using a wrist traction tower for distraction of the wrist during the procedure. A small joint arthroscope (2.3 mm) is used in the 3-4 portal for visualization of the TFCC tear, and the area is debrided and prepared in a standard fashion. Repair then involves placement of 2 or 3 sutures within the TFCC. Typically an absorbable, monofilament suture such as 2-0 polydioxanone (PDS) is used.

The outside-in technique originally described by de Araujo and colleagues[37] and modified by McAdams and colleagues[40] uses a 20-gauge Tuohy needle placed into the 3-4 portal or the 1-2 portal, allowing passage of suture in a radial to ulnar direction. The arthroscope is placed in the 6R portal to allow direct visualization of the repair. The needle is then passed through the torn TFCC peripheral rim and exits through a 1.5-cm longitudinal incision on the ulnar side of the wrist. Care must be taken to identify and protect the dorsal sensory branch of the ulnar nerve during needle passage and suture tying to decrease the chance of iatrogenic nerve injury. The needle trocar is then removed and a 2-0 PDS suture fed through the needle and out the ulnar incision. A small clamp secures the suture end on the ulnar side of the wrist and the needle is withdrawn back into the radiocarpal joint. The needle is then

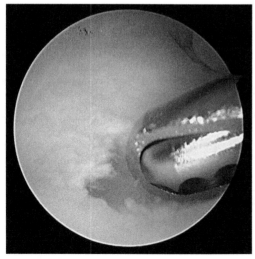

Fig. 5. Debridement of central TFCC tear.

advanced a few millimeters volar or dorsal and a second pass through the TFCC tear is performed. The beveled tip of the Tuohy needle will not cut the other limb of the suture, and allows it to be passed in the described fashion for creation of a horizontal mattress suture configuration or directly through the peripheral capsule in a simple suture configuration. The second suture end is then pulled through the needle, leaving 2 suture ends free on the ulnar side of the wrist to be tied under tension over the peripheral wrist capsule and ECU tendon subsheath. Traction should be removed from the wrist tower before tying the suture to take tension off the repair.

The outside-in repair, by contrast, is performed initially by creating a 1- to 1.5-cm incision just volar to the ECU tendon and distal to the ulnar styloid. The ECU tendon is retracted ulnarly and the dorsal branch of the ulnar nerve isolated and protected. A curved needle from a TFCC repair set is then placed through the ulnar capsule and into the torn TFCC. A straight needle is then inserted under direct arthroscopic visualization through the TFCC adjacent to the first and, using a wire loop, the suture end is retrieved and brought out through the ulnar incision and tied.

Results of arthroscopic repairs of Palmer 1B TFCC tears have been promising, with good to excellent results noted in 61% to 91% of patients in recent studies.[38,41–44] In a multicenter study, Corso and colleagues[38] found good to excellent results using an outside-in technique in 41 of 45 patients with an average follow-up of 37 months. The investigators noted that arthroscopic repair minimized soft-tissue trauma, improved appearance, and a led to a quicker recovery. Degreef and colleagues[41] noted significant pain relief in their cohort of patients, with 47 of 52 wrists presenting with minimal or absent pain. When lesser satisfactory outcome factors were analyzed, Ruch and Papadonikolakis[45] found a significant correlation with poorer outcomes and advancing age as well as ulnar-positive variance.

Literature has suggested that Type 1C and 1D TFCC tears are amenable to arthroscopic repair.[25,46,47] Trumble and colleagues[46] used an arthroscopic technique for the repair of radial-sided tears modified from that described by Cooney and colleagues[48] for open repairs. Using a standard 3-4 portal for visualization, the radial-sided tear is identified and the site on the radius for TFCC reattachment is debrided down to bleeding bone through the 6R portal using an arthroscopic shaver. A hypodermic needle is then placed into the ulnar aspect of the wrist just proximal to the triquetrum and the trajectory for suture repair introduction determined. A longitudinal stab incision following the needle path is then made, and an arthroscopic cannula placed into the wrist joint. Double-armed meniscal repair sutures are then passed through the cannula and into the radial edge of the TFCC. The sutures are then driven across the radius in a horizontal mattress pattern and exit the radial cortex between the first and second extensor compartments. The sutures are tied under tension with traction released and the wrist in neutral rotation.

Results of arthroscopic management of radial-sided lesions are limited. Trumble and colleagues[46] used the aforementioned technique for radial-sided tears in 13 patients. These investigators found improvement in grip strength and wrist range of motion of 89% and 87% that of the contralateral side, respectively. Eleven of 13 patients had complete relief of pain with all activities, whereas 2 had continued mild pain with moderate activity. Sagerman and Short[47] repaired radial-sided tears in a group of 12 patients, and at an average of 17 months yielded a 67% good or excellent clinical result. Specific data on objective outcome were not provided.

Open Repair

Open techniques for treatment of acute TFCC tears were the first established and validated treatment options for these injuries.[48] Cooney and colleagues[48] described an open technique using a dorsal ulnar incision in the interval between the fourth and fifth extensor compartments. After reflection of the extensor retinaculum, the ulnar carpal wrist capsule is incised in a line parallel to the direction of the TFCC. For radial-sided tears, an additional longitudinal incision is made in the DRUJ, proximal to the triangular fibrocartilage. This incision exposes the tear, and the location and extent can then be delineated with direct probing. The TFCC can then be repaired via drill holes placed within the dorsal aspect of the distal radius in a dorsoradial to palmar-ulnar direction, with the drill exiting at the edge of the junction between the lunate fossa and the sigmoid notch of the distal radius. Two or three 4-0 nylon horizontal mattress sutures are then placed into the TFCC and passed through the drill holes with a straight needle through bone. A reduction of the DRUJ is then performed by placing the forearm in a neutral to slight supination position. If alignment is suitable, the DRUJ is stabilized with 0.045-inch K-wires placed proximal to the joint, and the repair sutures tied over bone.

Using this technique in 33 patients, Cooney and colleagues[48] reported 11 excellent results, 15 good, 6 fair, and 1 poor result based on the Mayo Modified Wrist Score (MMWS). The average wrist score was 82 (range, 45–100). An associated ulnar recession was performed in 17 of the 33 patients. Anderson and colleagues[44] evaluated 39 patients treated with an open technique, and found 17 excellent and 9 good results (67%) based on the MMWS. The investigators also noted statistically significant improvements in pain and function on analysis of the MMWS.

Ruch and colleagues[49] performed a biomechanical cadaveric study comparing the strength of open TFCC repairs to the distal ulna using transosseous sutures through the fovea versus TFCC repairs to the ECU subsheath and dorsal ulnocarpal joint capsule. Six matched pairs of fresh frozen cadaveric upper extremities underwent each of the repairs using both extremities. Results showed a statistically significant improvement in DRUJ stability in both repair models. The mean percentage of total translation eliminated following repair in the transosseous group was 33.8% and in the capsular implantation group, 59.3%. The observed difference, however, was not statistically significant ($P = .157$).

Arthroscopic Versus Open Repair

The various arthroscopic TFCC tear repair techniques have emerged and gained popularity secondary to proponents claiming improved anatomic tear visualization, decreased injury to normal surrounding ulnar-sided wrist structures, and improved postoperative wrist motion.[23,47] However, the open repair technique is believed by many to be the only means by which the foveal connections of the TFCC can be anatomically restored.[50]

Only one study comparing the clinical outcomes of open and arthroscopic acute TFCC repair was found. Anderson and colleagues[44] performed a retrospective review of all patients who underwent TFCC tear repair surgery over a 10-year period. Seventy-five patients (36 treated arthroscopically and 39 treated with an open procedure) were included in the cohort with a mean average follow-up of 43 months. Pain and function improved as measured by the MMWS in both groups. No statistically significant differences in outcome scores were found between open and arthroscopic techniques. However, the investigators did note increased postoperative nerve pain (dorsal branch of ulnar nerve) as well as a slightly decreased clinical difference in postoperative wrist flexion/extension range of motion in the open group compared with the arthroscopic group, but both of these failed to reach statistical

significance as well. Anderson and colleagues also demonstrated a 17% reoperation rate for persistent DRUJ instability, with female patients having a 5-fold increase in the rate of reoperation.

SUMMARY

Injury to the TFCC is the most common cause of ulnar-sided wrist pain. Strategies for treatment of these injuries involve determining the anatomic location of the tear, the presence of associated DRUJ instability, and the presence of associated degenerative changes. Management of acute tears begins by defining the specific anatomic structures that have been disrupted, and treatment strategies are then matched to the injury. Surgical management with open and arthroscopic techniques have been described, both with successful results. Limited data exist, however, that compare functional outcomes.

REFERENCES

1. Palmer AK, Werner FW. The triangular fibrocartilage complex of the wrist- Anatomy and function. J Hand Surg Am 1981;6:153–62.
2. Stuart PR, Berger RA, Lischeid RL, et al. The dorsopalmar stability of the distal radioulnar joint. J Hand Surg Am 2000;25:689–99.
3. Kihara H, Short WH, Werner FW, et al. The stabilizing mechanism of the distal radioulnar joint during pronation and supination. J Hand Surg Am 1995; 20:930–6.
4. Watanabe H, Berger RA, Berglund LJ, et al. Contribution of the interosseous membrane to distal radioulnar joint constraint. J Hand Surg Am 2005;30: 1164–71.
5. Benjamin M, Evans EJ, Pemberton DJ. Histological studies on the triangular fibrocartilage complex of the wrist. J Anat 1990;172:59–67.
6. Bednar MS, Arnoczky SP, Weiland AJ. The microvasculature of the triangular fibrocartilage complex: its clinical significance. J Hand Surg Am 1991;16: 1101–5.
7. Boulas HJ, Milek MA. Ulnar shortening for tears of the triangular fibrocartilage complex. J Hand Surg Am 1990;15:415–20.
8. Hermansdorfer JD, Kleinman WB. Management of chronic peripheral tears of the triangular fibrocartilage complex. J Hand Surg Am 1991;16(2):340–6.
9. Minami A, Ishikawa J, Suenaga N, et al. Clinical results of treatment of triangular fibrocartilage complex tears by arthroscopic debridement. J Hand Surg Am 1996;21(3):406–11.
10. Tay SC, Tomita K, Berger RA. The "ulna fovea sign" for defining ulnar wrist pain: an analysis of sensitivity and specificity. J Hand Surg Am 2007;32:438–44.

11. Nagle DJ, Benson LS. Wrist arthroscopy: indications and results. Arthroscopy 1992;8:198–203.

12. Chung KC, Aimmerman NB, Travis MT. Wrist arthrography versus arthroscopy: a comparative study of 150 cases. J Hand Surg Am 1996;21:591–4.

13. Metz VM, Mann FA, Gilula LA. Lack of correlation between site of wrist pain and location of noncommunicating defects shown by three-compartment wrist arthrography. Am J Roentgenol 1993;160:1239–43.

14. Kirschenbaum D, Sieler S, Solonick D, et al. Arthrography of the wrist: assessment of the integrity of the ligaments in young asymptomatic adults. J Bone Joint Surg Am 1995;77:1207–9.

15. Herbert TJ, Faithfull RG, McCann DJ, et al. Bilateral arthrography of the wrist. J Hand Surg Br 1990;15:233–5.

16. Tanaka T, Yoshioka H, Ueno T, et al. Comparison between high-resolution MRI with a microscopy coil and arthroscopy in triangular fibrocartilage complex injury. J Hand Surg Am 2006;31:1308–14.

17. Saupe N, Prussmann KP, Luechinger R, et al. MR imaging of the wrist: comparison between 1.5 and 3 T MR imaging- preliminary experience. Radiology 2005;234:256–64.

18. Anderson ML, Skinner JA, Felmlee JP, et al. Diagnostic comparison of 1.5 Tesla and 3.0 Tesla preoperative MRI of the wrist in patients with ulnar-sided wrist pain. J Hand Surg Am 2008;33:1153–9.

19. Pederzini L, Luchetti R, Soragni O, et al. Evaluation of the triangular fibrocartilage complex tears by arthroscopy, arthrography and magnetic resonance imaging. Arthroscopy 1992;8:191–7.

20. Oneson SR, Timins ME, Scales LM, et al. MR imaging diagnosis of triangular fibrocartilage pathology with arthroscopic correlation. Am J Roentgenol 1997;168:1513–8.

21. Potter HG, Asnis-Ernberg L, Weiland AJ, et al. The utility of high-resolution magnetic resonance imaging in the evaluation of the triangular fibrocartilage complex of the wrist. J Bone Joint Surg Am 1997;79:1675–84.

22. Blazar PE, Chan PS, Kneeland JB, et al. The effect of observer experience on magnetic resonance imaging interpretation and localization of triangular fibrocartilage lesions. J Hand Surg Am 2001;26:742–8.

23. Bednar JM, Osterman AL. The role of arthroscopy in the treatment of traumatic triangular fibrocartilage injuries. Hand Clin 1994;10:605–14.

24. Nagle DJ. Arthroscopic treatment of degenerative tears of the triangular fibrocartilage. Hand Clin 1994;10:615–24.

25. Jantea CL, Baltzer A, Rüther W. Arthroscopic repair of radial-sided lesions of the triangular fibrocartilage complex. Hand Clin 1995;11:31–6.

26. Palmer AK. Triangular fibrocartilage complex lesions: a classification. J Hand Surg Am 1989;14:594–606.

27. Palmer AK, Werner FW, Glission RR, et al. Partial excision of the triangular fibrocartilage complex. J Hand Surg Am 1988;13:391–4.

28. Adams BD. Partial excision of the triangular fibrocartilage complex articular disk: a biomechanical study. J Hand Surg Am 1993;18:334–40.

29. Melone CP Jr, Nathan R. Traumatic disruption of the triangular fibrocartilage complex: pathoanatomy. Clin Orthop 1992;275:65–73.

30. Adams BD, Holley KA. Strains in the articular disk of the triangular fibrocartilage complex: a biomechanical study. J Hand Surg Am 1993;18:919–25.

31. Westkawmper JG, Mitsionis G, Giannakopoulous PN, et al. Wrist arthroscopy for the treatment of ligament and triangular fibrocartilage complex injuries. Arthroscopy 1998;14:479–83.

32. Whipple TL, Geissler WB. Arthroscopic management of wrist triangular fibrocartilage complex injuries in the athlete. Orthopedics 1993;16:1061–7.

33. Miwa H, Hashizume H, Fujiwara K, et al. Arthroscopic surgery for traumatic triangular fibrocartilage complex injury. J Orthop Sci 1994;9:354–9.

34. Blackwell RE, Jemison DM, Foy BD. The holmium:yttrium-aluminum garnet laser in wrist arthroscopy: a five-year experience in the treatment of central triangular fibrocartilage complex tears by partial excision. J Hand Surg Am 2001;26:77–84.

35. Bernstein MA, Nagle DJ, Martinez A, et al. A comparison of combined arthroscopic triangular fibrocartilage complex debridement and arthroscopic wafer distal ulna resection versus arthroscopic triangular fibrocartilage complex debridement and ulnar shortening osteotomy for ulnocarpal abutment syndrome. Arthroscopy 2004;20:392–401.

36. Hulsizer D, Weiss AP, Akelman E. Ulna-shortening osteotomy after failed arthroscopic debridement of the triangular fibrocartilage complex. J Hand Surg Am 1997;22A:694–8.

37. de Araujo W, Poehling GG, Kuzma GR. New Tuohy needle technique for triangular fibrocartilage complex repair: preliminary studies. Arthroscopy 1996;12:699–703.

38. Corso SJ, Savoie FH, Geissler WB, et al. Arthroscopic repair of peripheral avulsions of the triangular fibrocartilage complex of the wrist: a multicenter study. Arthroscopy 1997;13:78–84.

39. Böhringer G, Schadel-Höpfner M, Petermann J, et al. A method for all-inside arthroscopic repair of Palmer 1B triangular fibrocartilage complex tears. Arthroscopy 2002;18:211–3.

40. McAdams TR, Swan J, Yao J. Arthroscopic treatment of triangular fibrocartilage wrist injuries in the athlete. Am J Sports Med 2009;37:291–7.

41. Degreef I, Welters H, Milants P, et al. Disability and function after arthroscopic repair of ulnar avulsions

of the triangular fibrocartilage complex of the wrist. Acta Orthop Belg 2005;71:289–93.

42. Estrella EP, Hung LK, Ho PC, et al. Arthroscopic repair of triangular fibrocartilage complex tears. Arthroscopy 2007;23:729–37.

43. Millants P, De Smet L, Van Ransbeeck H. Outcome study of arthroscopic suturing of ulnar avulsions of the triangular fibrocartilage complex of the wrist. Chir Main 2002;21:298–300.

44. Anderson ML, Larson AN, Moran SL, et al. Clinical comparison of arthroscopic versus open repair of triangular fibrocartilage complex tears. J Hand Surg Am 2008;33A:675–82.

45. Ruch DS, Papadonikolakis A. Arthroscopically assisted repair of peripheral triangular fibrocartilage complex tears: factors affecting outcome. Arthroscopy 2005;21:1126–30.

46. Trumble TE, Gilbert M, Vedder N. Isolated tears of the triangular fibrocartilage: management by early arthroscopic repair. J Hand Surg Am 1997;22: 57–65.

47. Sagerman SD, Short W. Arthroscopic repair of radial-sided triangular fibrocartilage complex tears. Arthroscopy 1996;12:339–42.

48. Cooney WP, Linscheid RL, Dobyns JH. Triangular fibrocartilage tears. J Hand Surg Am 1994;19: 143–54.

49. Ruch DS, Anderson SR, Ritter MR. Biomechanical comparison of transosseous and capsular repair of peripheral triangular fibrocartilage tears. Arthroscopy 2003;19(4):391–6.

50. Trumble TE, Gilbert M, Vedder N. Arthroscopic repair of the triangular fibrocartilage complex. Arthroscopy 1996;12:588–97.

Longitudinal Split Tears of the Ulnotriquetral Ligament

Shian-Chao Tay, MD, MS[a,b], Richard A. Berger, MD, PhD[c],*,
Wendy L. Parker, MD, PhD[d]

KEYWORDS

- Ulnotriquetral ligament • Ulnar sided wrist pain
- Longitudinal split tears • Triangular fibrocartilage complex

The complexity of soft tissue anatomy on the ulnar side of the wrist has made agreement regarding what constitutes normal anatomy difficult.[1–6] In addition, the large number of structures that can be injured in the ulnar wrist and the likelihood that they serve their function in a synergistic manner, make the examination and study of injuries in this region difficult. Multiple diagnoses can be made; they include peripheral tears of the triangular fibrocartilage complex (TFCC), foveal avulsions, lunotriquetral ligament injuries, extensor carpi ulnaris (ECU) tendon and subsheath pathologies, and ulnar styloid impaction,[7] just to name a few. As such, ulnar sided wrist pain continues to be a "black box" and is often considered the "low-back pain" in hand surgery.[8]

The purpose of this article is to describe the cause of chronic ulnar wrist pain arising from a longitudinal split tear of the ulnotriquetral (UT) ligament. Unlike tears of the peripheral triangular fibrocartilage (TFC) or avulsions of the distal radioulnar ligaments, longitudinal split tears of the UT ligament do not cause any instability to the distal radioulnar joint or the ulnocarpal articulation. It is mainly a pain syndrome that can be incapacitating. However, because the UT ligament arises from the palmar radioulnar (PRU) ligament of the TFCC, it is by definition, an injury of the TFCC. According to Palmer classification, this injury is a form of type IC injury that has not been previously described.[9]

ANATOMY

The PRU and dorsal radioulnar (DRU) ligaments are the primary ligamentous stabilizers of the distal radioulnar joint. The PRU and the DRU ligaments arise from the palmar and dorsal edge of the sigmoid notch, respectively. Both the ligaments converge ulnarly and interdigitate for a strong attachment to the fovea of the ulna head. From there, some of the conjoined fibers of the PRU and DRU ligaments also insert into the styloid process of the ulna.[10] The interval between the PRU and DRU ligaments is spanned by a sheet of fibrocartilage known as the TFC. The TFC together with the PRU and DRU ligaments forms the TFCC. The DRU ligament splits ulnarly to form part of the subretinacular sheath for the ECU tendon (**Fig. 1**). As such, the ECU subsheath is attached to the ulnar styloid and the ulnar fovea through the DRU ligament.[2,4,5,11]

The PRU ligament forms the proximal attachment of the ulnolunate (UL) and UT

The authors have nothing to disclose.

[a] Orthopedic Surgery, Mayo Clinic College of Medicine, 200th First Street South West, Rochester, MN 55905, USA
[b] Division of Hand Surgery, Singapore General Hospital, Singapore
[c] Division of Hand Surgery, Department of Orthopaedic Surgery, Mayo Clinic, 200 1st Street SW, Rochester, MN 55905, USA
[d] Department of Surgery Scott and White Clinic, Texas A&M University, Temple, TX, USA
* Corresponding author.
E-mail address: berger.richard@mayo.edu

Hand Clin 26 (2010) 495–501
doi:10.1016/j.hcl.2010.07.004
0749-0712/10/$ — see front matter © 2010 Elsevier Inc. All rights reserved.

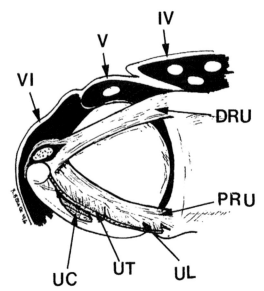

Fig. 1. As seen from a distal perspective, the DRU ligament splits to form the ECU tendon subsheath, which is deep to the sixth extensor compartment (VI). The PRU ligament provides the origin for the ulnolunate (UL) and ulnotriquetral (UT) ligaments. The ulnocapitate (UC) ligament, however, is more superficial and has a direct bony attachment to the fovea of the ulnar head. (*From* Berger RA. The ligaments of the wrist. A current overview of anatomy with considerations of their potential functions. Hand Clin 1997;13(1):68, Fig 2; with permission.)

ligaments.[2,4,5,11] The UL ligament arises from the PRU ligament and inserts distally into the lunate on its proximal and palmar margins. The UT ligament has a more oblique orientation than the UL ligament. UT ligament arises from the PRU ligament, ulnar to the UL ligament, and the palmar radial aspect of the base of the ulnar styloid.[1,5,6] Distally, the UT ligament attaches to the palmar and ulnar aspects of the triquetrum.[4,5] Arthroscopically, there is no clear demarcation between the UL and UT ligaments. The distinction between the 2 ligaments can only be made by their distal attachments.[5]

The UT ligament often contains 2 perforations, the prestyloid recess and the pisotriquetral orifice.[5] Arthroscopically, the prestyloid recess was found to be located at the ulnar junction between the PRU and UT ligaments.[11] Just distal and anterior to the prestyloid recess and anterior to the proximal articular surface of the triquetrum, is the pisotriquetral orifice, which is present in 90% of normal individuals.[11]

The third ligament of the ulnocarpal complex is the ulnocapitate (UC) ligament. Unlike the UL and UT ligaments, the UC ligament does not arise from the PRU ligament. From an extra-articular

perspective, the UC ligament is superficial and arises directly from the foveal region of the distal ulna bone (see **Fig. 1**). It travels distally, anterior to the junction of the UL and UT ligaments, until it reaches the lunotriquetral joint (**Fig. 2**), where it reinforces the palmar lunotriquetral ligament before interdigitating with the fibers of the radioscaphocapitate ligament at the midcarpal joint.[5]

INJURY MECHANISM

In a retrospective review by the senior author (R.A.B.), 36 patients with longitudinal split tears of the UT ligament were studied. Of them, 23 patients (64%) reported a single traumatic event preceding their symptoms, with 4 patients (11%) reporting histories consistent with repetitive trauma. No history of memorable trauma was elicited in the remaining 9 patients (15%). Of the 27 patients who reported a history of trauma, single or repetitive occurrence, 26 patients (96%) reported a mechanism of injury that involved wrist hyperextension and forearm supination.

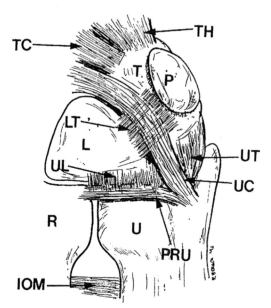

Fig. 2. The palmar ulnocarpal ligaments from a palmar perspective. The UC ligament has a direct bony origin from the fovea of the ulnar head, is more superficial, and is anterior to the junction between the UL and UT ligaments. Both the UL and UT ligaments originate from the PRU ligament. The UC ligament reinforces the palmar LT ligament distally. IOM, interosseous membrane; L, lunate; LT, lunotriquetral; P, pisiform; R, radius; T, triquetrum; TC, triquetrocapitate; TH, triquetrohamate; U, ulna. (*From* Berger RA. The ligaments of the wrist. A current overview of anatomy with considerations of their potential functions. Hand Clin 1997;13(1):73, Fig 11; with permission.)

Biomechanical studies on the UT ligament have shown that its length is maximum during wrist radial extension,[12] a combination of maximal wrist extension and radial deviation. This extension seems to be equivalent to the extension phase of the dart-throw motion in the wrist.[13] In addition, the tension in the UT ligament was shown to be higher during supination than pronation.[14]

Moritomo and colleagues[12] suggested that excessive traction of the ulnocarpal ligaments, caused by hyper-radial extension or hyperextension of the wrist combined with axial loading or forearm rotation (or both), could transmit forces down to the ulnar fovea and cause avulsions of the TFCC, thus producing Palmer type IB injuries. According to the authors, forces experienced by the ligament approaching, but not reaching those required to produce a foveal tear, could also produce a split tear of the UT ligament.

Based on the authors' clinical data and the above-mentioned biomechanical studies, the authors think that a combination of axial loading of the hand, radial extension of the wrist, and supination of the forearm puts the UT ligament in a situation in which it is subjected to maximum traction. In this situation, the ligament experiences concomitant longitudinal traction (from radial extension and forearm supination) and countertorsion (forearm supination).

As to why the ligament splits instead of tearing or avulsing during traction, the authors think that 2 factors may play a part. First, the UT ligament may contain a longitudinal zone of relative weakness because of the presence of the prestyloid recess and the pisotriquetral orifice. Second, the foveal attachment of the UT ligament, via the PRU ligament, may be stronger than the ulnar styloid attachment of the UT ligament.[10] When the UT ligament is subjected to excessive traction, the ulnar styloid attachment may fail before the foveal attachment, thus resulting in the ligament splitting at the interface between the fibers that insert into the PRU ligament and the ulnar styloid **(Fig. 3)**.

PATIENT PROFILE

Based on the review of the 36 patients, the average age of a patient with a longitudinal split tear of the UT ligament was 30 years, with a range of 14 to 70 years. About half of the patients were men and one-third were athletes. All 36 patients had a chief complaint of ulnar sided wrist pain with 70% of the complaints being on the right wrist. The average duration of symptoms was 14.9 months, with a range of 14 days to 6 years.

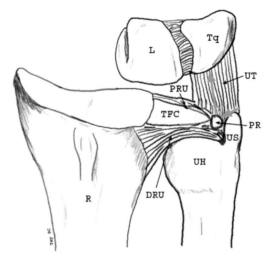

Fig. 3. When subjected to a combination of loading, wrist extension/radial extension, and forearm supination the UT ligament experiences conditions of maximal traction. This condition may cause the ulnar styloid fibers to detach early (*horizontal red arrow*). The ligament injury then propagates along the path of weakness found between the PR and the pisotriquetral orifice (*vertical red arrow*), thus producing a longitudinal split tear of the UT ligament. L, lunate; PR, prestyloid recess; R, radius; Tq, triquetrum; UH, ulnar head; US, ulnar styloid. (*Adapted from* Sasao S, Beppu M, Kihara H, et al. An anatomical study of the ligaments of the ulnar compartment of the wrist. Hand Surg 2003;8(2):219–26. p. 221, Fig. 1a; with permission.)

All patients reported worsening of pain with gripping. Most patients (80%) also reported worsening of pain with forearm supination and pronation. Worsening of pain can occur with or without concomitant heavy lifting. Most (72%) of the patients had sought medical treatment previously and have not responded to either conservative or surgical treatment.

DIAGNOSIS

A comprehensive wrist examination should be performed in all cases. Grip strength should be measured and will be found to be decreased. Range of motion of the wrist, including forearm pronation and supination, should also be documented. In patients with isolated UT split tears, range of motion is normal. If forearm rotation is found to be abnormal, the problem may be elsewhere, such as in the distal radioulnar joint. Point tenderness in the wrist should also be evaluated in the normal fashion.

The key clinical test for the diagnosis of longitudinal split tear of the UT ligament is to detect the presence or absence of ulnar fovea tenderness, also known as the "ulnar fovea sign."[15] The ulnar fovea sign is a provocative maneuver aimed at eliciting abnormal tenderness in the ulnar fovea. This sign is elicited with the patient sitting with his or her elbow on the table opposite the examiner. The patient's upper limb should be relaxed, and the examiner should support the patient's hand to keep the elbow in 90° to 110° of flexion with the wrist in neutral rotation. The forearm must be in neutral rotation. The examiner then presses his or her thumb tip distally and deep into the interval "soft spot" between the ulnar styloid process, flexor carpi ulnaris tendon, volar surface of the ulnar head, and the pisiform (**Figs. 4** and **5**). The ulnar fovea sign is positive when there is exquisite tenderness compared with the contralateral side. Typically, this tenderness replicates the patient's complaint of pain in terms of character and location. The context of the clinical sign is important, and the clinical sign is most useful in a symptomatic patient who has no other obvious evidence of pathology in the wrist. As such, this clinical sign is not as useful in cases in which the patient has global tenderness of the wrist.

Once a positive ulnar fovea sign is elicited, stability of the distal radioulnar joint must be

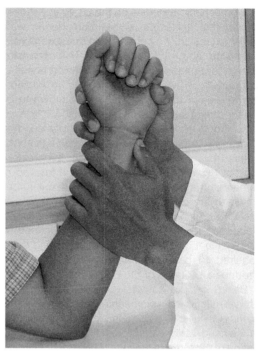

Fig. 5. The detection of ulnar fovea sign must be performed with the forearm in neutral rotation. The wrist must also be in neutral rotation without any flexion or extension. The patient should be asked to relax the upper limb. The examiner should support the patient's hand while using his or her thumb tip to press into the fovea region.

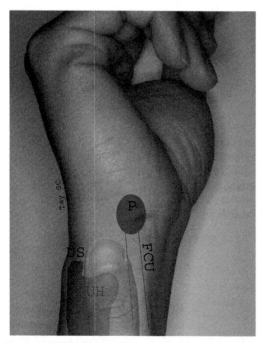

Fig. 4. With the forearm in neutral rotation, the fovea region is bound dorsally by the ulnar styloid (US), proximally by the curved surface of the ulnar head (UH), volarly by the flexor carpi ulnaris (FCU) tendon, and distally by the pisiform (P). The semitransparent thumb tip of the examiner is shown pressing into the fovea region.

determined. If the distal radioulnar joint is stable, the diagnosis of longitudinal split tear of the UT ligament can be made. If the distal radioulnar joint is found to be unstable, foveal avulsion of the TFCC, a Palmer type IB lesion, should be suspected (**Fig. 6**).

In a validation study, it was found that a positive ulnar fovea sign was 95% sensitive and 87% specific in the clinical detection of foveal avulsions and/or longitudinal split tears of the UT ligament. In patients with clinically stable distal radioulnar joint, a positive ulnar fovea sign was 90% sensitive and 88% specific in detecting longitudinal split tears of the UT ligament.[15]

Wrist radiographs are usually noncontributory to the diagnosis of longitudinal split tears of the UT ligament. High-resolution magnetic resonance imaging (MRI) may be potentially helpful in detecting UT ligament injuries. In the 36 patients with longitudinal split tears of the UT ligament, 30 underwent MRI of the wrist. Signal changes consistent with fluid accumulation were demonstrated in the substance of the UT ligament (10 patients), in the foveal insertion of the TFCC (9 patients), and in both the structures (3 patients).

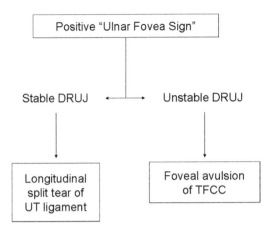

Fig. 6. A positive ulnar fovea sign is sensitive and specific for 2 conditions: longitudinal split tear of the UT ligament and foveal avulsion of the TFCC. The differentiation between the 2 conditions can be made clinically by determining the stability of the distal radioulnar joint (DRUJ).

Aside from signal changes, no specific MRI features have been found that can be used to specifically diagnose a longitudinal split tear of the UT ligament.[16]

Arthroscopy

At present, wrist arthroscopy is the only way to confirm a diagnosis of longitudinal split tear of the UT ligament. The pathologic condition is typically viewed from the 3-4 portal and is identified first as a region of proliferative synovial villi, extending from the prestyloid recess toward the pisotriquetral joint (**Fig. 7**). Once the synovial villi are debrided, a longitudinal defect within the substance of the UT ligament is evident (**Fig. 8**). The inner longitudinal fibers of the UT ligament can be seen on either side of the defect. Providing external pressure using the thumb tip in the ulnar fovea region should displace the UT ligament and in some cases, apposes the longitudinal fibers, giving the appearance of closing the defect.

OPERATIVE PROCEDURE

The surgery can be performed under general or regional anesthesia. An arm tourniquet should be placed before surgery and can be inflated intraoperatively to assist in hemostasis. Wrist arthroscopy can be performed using scopes measuring from 1.9 mm to 2.7 mm. Radiocarpal portals that can be used include the 3-4, 4-5, or 6R portals. Midcarpal portals, when indicated, include the radial and ulnar midcarpal portals.

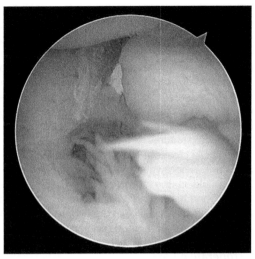

Fig. 7. The region of the longitudinal split tear of the UT ligament is initially concealed by synovial villi proliferation, extending from the prestyloid recess toward the pisotriquetral joint.

As part of standard arthroscopic examination, the stability of the TFC should be determined using a probe and the trampoline sign assessed. The integrity of the foveal attachment of the DRU and PRU ligaments is verified by hooking the TFCC at the prestyloid recess and attempting to displace the TFCC distally. If the TFCC is stable and the longitudinal split tear of the UT ligament is the primary pathology, the longitudinal split tear should be repaired using an "outside-to-inside" repair.[17]

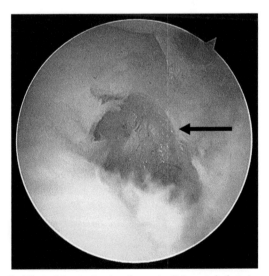

Fig. 8. Arthroscopic view from the 3-4 portal, showing the longitudinal split tear of the UT ligament (*arrow*) after debridement of the synovial villi.

The outside-to-inside repair is performed by first making a 1-cm longitudinal incision just anterior to the ECU tendon, starting distal to the ulnar styloid process. The dorsal sensory branch of the ulnar nerve is identified deep to the basilic vein and should be protected. Using the Meniscus Mender II suture system, 1 or 2 lengths of 2-0 polydioxanone sutures are passed across the split tear using the standard outside-to-inside suture technique. When these sutures are tied, the split tear is anatomically closed (**Fig. 9**). Arthroscopic instruments are withdrawn at the end of the procedure, excess fluid in the subcutaneous tissue is expressed, and the wounds are closed. The forearm should then be held in a sugar-tong splint that holds the forearm in neutral rotation.

Postoperative Care

The surgical dressing is removed at the first postoperative visit. Sutures can be removed at 10 to 14 days postoperation. The sugar-tong plaster splint is replaced with an above-elbow cast while maintaining the forearm in neutral rotation for 6 weeks. After this period, a Muenster-type splint is used with the forearm in neutral rotation. At this time, the patient is educated on home-based active range of motion exercises for forearm and wrist range of motion and instructed to reduce splint use and increase activities as tolerated with no specific restrictions enforced. No formal ongoing therapy is required. Patients are usually followed up for 4 to 5 months postoperation and are advised to return only if there is persistent pain or other concerns.

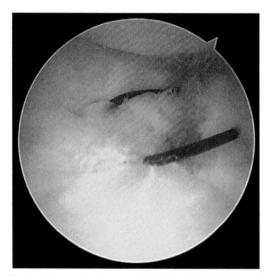

Fig. 9. Anatomic closure of the longitudinal tear of the UT ligament is achieved using 2 strands of 2-0 polydioxanone sutures.

OUTCOMES

In the series of patients studied by the senior author, the satisfaction rate was 89%. Overall, 90% of patients reported no limitations of activity whatsoever. Preoperatively, mean grip strength was 31 kg and 38 kg on the affected and contralateral sides, respectively. Postoperative grip strength was a mean of 33 kg and 40 kg on the affected and contralateral sides, respectively. The difference in range of motion of the wrist preoperatively and postoperatively was statistically not significant.

The average disabilities of the arm, shoulder and hand score at 28.2 months postoperation was 7.5 (SD 9.8) overall, with 4.9 for work-related section and 7.6 for sports/music related section. Improved scores were seen in men, laborers, and older age groups. Using the patient-rated wrist evaluation,[18] patients scored a mean of 14.8 out of a possible 150 points, which corresponds to a minimal disability rating.

There were no intraoperative or postoperative complications. However, 2 of the 36 patients eventually underwent formal distal radioulnar joint ligament reconstruction using a free tendon graft.[19] One of the 2 patients had mild distal radioulnar joint instability with some laxity of the TFCC during the arthroscopic UT ligament repair. This instability probably indicated that there was a partial avulsion of the foveal attachment; however, it was not severe enough to require any further reconstructive surgery at that time, and only the UT ligament was repaired. This patient subsequently developed progressive multidirectional instability of the distal radioulnar joint and underwent reconstruction 33.5 months later. The second patient had recovered well from the UT repair surgery and was satisfied, returning to play baseball. However, this patient sustained a new injury 7 weeks later and had to undergo ligament reconstruction 5 months later.

SUMMARY

The detection of ulnar fovea sign is an important test in the clinical evaluation of ulnar sided wrist pain. The sign indicates 2 conditions: a longitudinal split tear of the UT ligament or foveal avulsion of the TFCC. The discrimination between the 2 conditions is decided by the presence or absence of distal radioulnar joint instability. Although a positive ulnar fovea sign without distal radioulnar joint instability is a strong predictor of longitudinal split tears of the UT ligament, at present, wrist arthroscopy remains the gold standard for the diagnosis and treatment of this condition.

This article has described in detail a novel injury to the TFCC, the longitudinal split tear of the UT ligament, and a clinical test, detection of the ulnar fovea sign. The consistency in mechanism of injury, symptoms, and arthroscopic findings confirms this injury as a true pathologic condition. The senior author's early experience in treating these lesions with simple arthroscopic debridement without suture repair led to substantially inferior results. The outside-to-inside repair method demonstrates convincing patient outcomes and high patient satisfaction rate.

The authors propose that a modification to the Palmer 1C classification be made to include: (1) transverse or avulsion injuries of the ulnocarpal ligaments and (2) longitudinal split tears of the UT ligament.

REFERENCES

1. Ishii S, Palmer AK, Werner FW, et al. An anatomic study of the ligamentous structure of the triangular fibrocartilage complex. J Hand Surg Am 1998;23(6): 977–85.

2. Nakamura T, Yabe Y. Histological anatomy of the triangular fibrocartilage complex of the human wrist. Ann Anat 2000;182(6):567–72.

3. Nakamura T, Yabe Y, Horiuchi Y. Functional anatomy of the triangular fibrocartilage complex. J Hand Surg Br 1996;21(5):581–6.

4. Berger RA. The ligaments of the wrist. A current overview of anatomy with considerations of their potential functions. Hand Clin 1997;13(1):63–82.

5. Berger RA. The anatomy of the ligaments of the wrist and distal radioulnar joints. Clin Orthop Relat Res 2001;383:32–40.

6. Sasao S, Beppu M, Kihara H, et al. An anatomical study of the ligaments of the ulnar compartment of the wrist. Hand Surg 2003;8(2):219–26.

7. Topper SM, Wood MB, Ruby LK. Ulnar styloid impaction syndrome. J Hand Surg Am 1997;22(4):699–704.

8. Shin AY, Deitch MA, Sachar K, et al. Ulnar-sided wrist pain: diagnosis and treatment. Instr Course Lect 2005;54:115–28.

9. Palmer AK. Triangular fibrocartilage complex lesions: a classification. J Hand Surg Am 1989;14(4): 594–606.

10. Haugstvedt JR, Berger RA, Nakamura T, et al. Relative contributions of the ulnar attachments of the triangular fibrocartilage complex to the dynamic stability of the distal radioulnar joint. J Hand Surg Am 2006;31(3):445–51.

11. Berger RA. Arthroscopic anatomy of the wrist and distal radioulnar joint. Hand Clin 1999;15(3): 393–413, vii.

12. Moritomo H, Murase T, Arimitsu S, et al. Change in the length of the ulnocarpal ligaments during radiocarpal motion: possible impact on triangular fibrocartilage complex foveal tears. J Hand Surg Am 2008;33(8):1278–86.

13. Wolfe SW, Crisco JJ, Orr CM, et al. The dart-throwing motion of the wrist: is it unique to humans? J Hand Surg Am 2006;31(9):1429–37.

14. DiTano O, Trumble TE, Tencer AF. Biomechanical function of the distal radioulnar and ulnocarpal wrist ligaments. J Hand Surg Am 2003;28(4): 622–7.

15. Tay SC, Tomita K, Berger RA. The "ulnar fovea sign" for defining ulnar wrist pain: an analysis of sensitivity and specificity. J Hand Surg Am 2007;32(4): 438–44.

16. Anderson ML, Skinner JA, Felmlee JP, et al. Diagnostic comparison of 1.5 Tesla and 3.0 Tesla preoperative MRI of the wrist in patients with ulnar-sided wrist pain. J Hand Surg Am 2008;33(7):1153–9.

17. Whipple TL, Geissler WB. Arthroscopic management of wrist triangular fibrocartilage complex injuries in the athlete. Orthopedics 1993;16(9): 1061–7.

18. John M, Angst F, Awiszus F, et al. The patient-rated wrist evaluation (PRWE): cross-cultural adaptation into German and evaluation of its psychometric properties. Clin Exp Rheumatol 2008;26(6): 1047–58.

19. Adams BD, Berger RA. An anatomic reconstruction of the distal radioulnar ligaments for posttraumatic distal radioulnar joint instability. J Hand Surg Am 2002;27(2):243–51.

Acute Dislocations of the Distal Radioulnar Joint and Distal Ulna Fractures

Brian T. Carlsen, MD[a,b], David G. Dennison, MD[b], Steven L. Moran, MD[a,b],*

KEYWORDS

- Distal radioulnar joint • Dislocation
- Ulna fractures • Wrist trauma

ANATOMY AND BIOMECHANICS OF THE DISTAL RADIOULNAR JOINT

The ulna is the fixed unit of the forearm joint, with the hand, carpus, and radius rotating around it.[1] Rotational forearm motion occurs at the distal radioulnar joint (DRUJ) and proximal radioulnar joint (PRUJ) at the elbow. DRUJ motion is primarily rotational, but there are components of axial and translational motion that occur during loading and rotation. Axial motion is due to the crossing relationship of the radius to the ulna in pronation. This axial motion can produce changes in the ulnar variance that may be as great as 2 mm with full forearm rotation.[2–5] Dorsal and palmar translational motion of the radius about the fixed ulnar head also occurs with supination and pronation, respectively.[6–8]

Joint stability at the DRUJ is provided through a combination of bony architecture and soft tissue constraints, which include the ligaments found in the triangular fibrocartilage complex (TFCC), the pronator quadratus, and the interosseous membrane (IOM). The bony architecture of the DRUJ accounts for only 20% of the joint's stability[9]; thus most of the stability is provided by the soft tissue attachments. In addition, individual variation in the bony configuration of the DRUJ may also affect its stability. A study by Tolat and

colleagues[10] defined the shape of the sigmoid notch in the transverse plane in 4 different configurations: flat face (42% incidence), ski slope (14%), C-type (30%), and S-type (14%). Although the study did not include biomechanical evaluation of the different joint configurations, the investigators proposed that this may have important implications in the bony contribution to joint stability.[10]

The primary stabilizer of the DRUJ is the TFCC, originally described by Palmer and Werner.[11] The TFCC is composed of several structures, including the triangular fibrocartilage (TFC), the ulnocarpal meniscus (meniscus homolog), the ulnar collateral ligament, the dorsal radioulnar ligament, the palmar radioulnar ligament, and the subsheath of the extensor carpi ulnaris (ECU).[11] These structures are not readily distinguishable on anatomic dissection and together are referred to as the TFCC. The central portion of the TFC makes up the articular disk. This disk forms the ulnocarpal articulation and effectively cushions the ulnar head. In contrast to the peripheral TFCC, the articular disk is relatively avascular and therefore is presumed to be incapable of significant healing capabilities.[12]

The dorsal and palmar radioulnar ligaments are thought to be responsible for most of the stability at the DRUJ.[9,13] Significant research has been performed to determine which component of the

[a] Division of Plastic Surgery, Department of Surgery, Mayo Clinic, 200 First Street SW, Rochester, MN 55905, USA
[b] Division of Hand Surgery, Department of Orthopaedic Surgery, Mayo Clinic, 200 First Street SW, Rochester, MN 55905, USA
* Corresponding author. Division of Hand Surgery, Department of Orthopaedic Surgery, Mayo Clinic, 200 First Street SW, Rochester, MN 55905.
E-mail address: moran.steven@mayo.edu

Hand Clin 26 (2010) 503–516
doi:10.1016/j.hcl.2010.05.009
0749-0712/10/$ – see front matter © 2010 Elsevier Inc. All rights reserved.

radioulnar ligament complex (palmar or dorsal) is more critical for joint stability.[14–16] Hagert,[13] in 1994, helped answer this question and recognized that palmar and dorsal components of the radioulnar ligaments were necessary for DRUJ stability. Hagert described the existence of superficial and deep portions of the the dorsal and palmar radioulnar ligaments. The superficial fibers attach to the base of the ulnar styloid and thus are susceptible to injury in cases of peripheral TFCC tears. The deep fibers, sometimes referred to as the ligamentum subcruentum, attach to the fovea and are thus susceptible to injury in cases of basilar ulnar styloid fractures. In pronation, the dorsal superficial fibers tighten together with the palmar deep fibers. Conversely, in supination, the palmar superficial fibers together with the dorsal deep fibers are taut and effectively constrain DRUJ motion.[13] Other studies have confirmed the reciprocal relationship between the superficial and deep portions of the radioulnar ligament, further emphasizing that the deep palmar and dorsal ligaments attach to the fovea and prevent dorsal and palmar subluxation with forearm rotation, respectively. The superficial palmar and dorsal ligaments attach to the ulnar styloid and act as rotational restraints to supination and pronation, respectively.[17,18] Work by Stuart and colleagues[9] and other investigators have shown that dorsal displacement of the distal ulna relative to the radius is most likely because of failure of the palmar radioulnar ligament, whereas palmar displacement of the ulna relative to the radius is because of failure of the dorsal radioulnar ligament.[19–21]

An additional secondary constraint to palmar displacement and dislocation includes the IOM.[16,22–24] The IOM contains several ligamentous components along its length. The central band is a stout ligament that runs obliquely from proximal on the radius to distal on the ulna, fanning out towards its insertion on the ulna.[25] The central band is thought to play an important role in the longitudinal stabilization of the forearm.[25,26] The distal oblique bundle is a thick band of tissue in the distal one-sixth of the membrane. It originates proximally on the ulnar shaft, in the same location as the proximal pronator quadratus muscle, and attaches distally to the capsule of the DRUJ. The bundle may contribute some fibers to the volar and dorsal radioulnar ligaments.[23] Although this structure is consistently present, its thickness may vary from patient to patient.[22,23]

Acute Isolated DRUJ Dislocation

As previously mentioned, the ulna is the fixed structure of the forearm, and anatomically it is the radius that dislocates away from its original anatomic position. However, the clinical and radiographic appearance of DRUJ dislocation is one of ulnar dislocation relative to the radius, which has resulted in the historic description of such injuries in terms of the ulna's relationship to the radius. In this article, the authors use this technically incorrect but widely accepted description. They refer to a dorsal dislocation as occurring when the ulna resides dorsal to the radius and volar dislocation as occurring when the ulna resides volar to the radius.

Isolated acute dislocation of the DRUJ (with or without ulnar styloid fracture) is less common than dislocation associated with a fracture of the radius or distal ulna.[27] The first report of an isolated dislocation of the DRUJ without fracture was by Desault in 1777.[28,29] Since then, there have been numerous case reports and small series describing such injuries.[6,19,30–35] The direction of dislocation can be either volar or dorsal, although dorsal dislocation is probably more common.

Dorsal dislocations are believed to result from a hyperpronation force, and volar dislocations from a hypersupination force.[19–21] Although an acute dislocation must result in an injury to the TFCC, the amount and degree of injury required for dislocation of the DRUJ is not entirely clear and DRUJ dislocation may not require complete disruption of the TFCC.[19,32,36,37] One premise for this observation is that, in many cases, the DRUJ is notably stable after reduction of the dislocation.[6,32] Hagert[13,38] has described injury of the volar radioulnar ligament and dorsal joint capsule with dorsal dislocation. The reverse mechanism also occurs with rupture of the dorsal radioulnar ligament and volar joint capsule in a volar dislocation.[36]

In a dorsal dislocation, there is typically a history of hyperpronation force, usually as a result of a fall on the outstretched hand. In this situation, the hand is typically fixed by gravity to the ground, and the body, together with the ulna, rotates around the hand, wrist, and radius unit. The patient presents with the hand fixed in pronation, with the inability to supinate and a dorsal prominence of the ulnar head.

In cases of volar dislocation, there is a history of hypersupination and the patient is unable to pronate. The ulnar head is usually not visibly prominent on the volar wrist because of the overlying soft tissues. However, there can be a hollow dorsally where the ulnar head is usually visible in the uninjured wrist. The wrist can appear narrow because of the now compressive pull of the pronator quadratus muscle, resulting in a diminished transverse dimension.[29,36] In either direction of dislocation, the examination findings can be obscured by ecchymosis and swelling.

Plain 2-view radiographs that include the wrist, forearm, and elbow are critical for the evaluation of suspected DRUJ dislocation. The anteroposterior (AP) view in a dorsal dislocation typically shows a widened DRUJ with divergence of the radius and ulna when compared with the contralateral normal DRUJ, whereas a volar dislocation demonstrates an overlap of the radius and ulna at the DRUJ because of the convergent pull of the pronator quadratus. In an anatomically reduced DRUJ in neutral rotation, the ulnar styloid is located at the most medial (ulnar) aspect of the ulnar head. A standard posteroanterior view of the wrist is taken with the shoulder abducted 90° and the elbow at 90° flexion and neutral forearm rotation. This view is often not possible in the setting of acute DRUJ dislocation because of mechanical blockage caused by the dislocation, pain, or splint immobilization, and unfortunately, oblique films are obtained more often than true orthogonal radiographs. Therefore, one must be careful in the interpretation of these radiographs. As little as a 10° obliquely malaligned view of a dislocation may appear to be reduced and thus falsely interpreted as negative.[39] One valuable criterion in determining a true lateral radiograph is the scaphopisocapitate alignment.[40] In this analysis, the volar cortex of the pisiform overlies the central third of the interval between the volar cortices of the distal pole of the scaphoid and the capitate head, confirming a true lateral view.[40] An axial computed tomographic (CT) scan may be helpful in the acute setting to determine joint reduction and congruity.[39,41] Various measures have been described to evaluate for translation at the DRUJ, with the subluxation ratio method being the most reliable in terms of intra- and interobserver reliability.[42]

Treatment of acute DRUJ dislocations

Treatment of the acute dislocation without fracture begins with closed reduction. This treatment is typically accomplished under local anesthesia with or without sedation. In dorsal dislocations of the ulna, reduction is accomplished with gentle traction, dorsal pressure (translational force) over the ulnar head, and supination. The joint must be assessed for instability and typically is most stable in supination. In volar dislocations, reduction can be more difficult because of the pull of the pronator quadratus muscle. To achieve reduction, one may have to distract the ulna from the radius (or vice versa) in conjunction with the volar pressure (translational force) over the ulnar head and pronation. Regional or general anesthesia may

be necessary to achieve closed reduction. Because of the vascularity and healing potential of the peripheral TFCC,[12] closed treatment is frequently successful in the restoration of a stable construct.

So-called complex dislocations occur when there is interposed soft tissue that blocks closed reduction. These dislocations typically occur in conjunction with a Galeazzi fracture and are discussed later; however, nonreducible simple dislocations without soft tissue interposition can also occur. In such a case, the ulna may be irreducible because of a bony mechanical blockage at the volar lip of the sigmoid notch of the radius (**Fig. 1**).[43] If it is necessary to perform open reduction, then direct repair of the TFCC to the foveal insertion is preferred. The procedure is performed using suture anchors or heavy suture through bone tunnels. Although this is the authors' preference, they know of no studies demonstrating improved outcomes over reduction and immobilization in this situation. A study by Ruch and colleagues[44] looked at patients with distal radius fractures and DRUJ instability with a large, displaced ulnar styloid fragment. The 2 treatment groups consisted of (1) open treatment with tension band fixation and (2) DRUJ immobilization with an ulnar outrigger in 60° supination. The investigators found a tendency toward improved supination

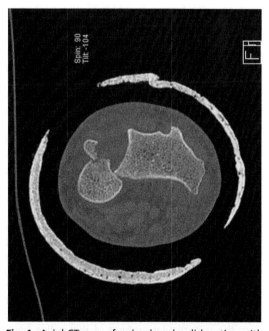

Fig. 1. Axial CT scan of a simple volar dislocation with ulnar styloid fracture. The dislocation required open reduction because of the mechanical blockage of the volar lip of the sigmoid notch.

and fewer DRUJ-related complications in the group of patients treated with the external fixator.[44] After TFCC repair, the forearm can be immobilized in a long-arm or Munster-type cast with or without transcutaneous radioulnar pinning. The authors' preference is to place two 0.062-in Kirschner (K) wires just proximal to the DRUJ obtaining purchase of 4 cortices and leaving the wires slightly prominent on the radial and ulnar superficial cortices, which allows for easy wire removal should one or both pins break between the radius and ulna. The authors prefer immobilization in neutral rotation to facilitate recovery of pronation and supination after the period of immobilization. Alternatively, the forearm is immobilized in the position of maximal stability, supination for dorsal dislocations and pronation for volar dislocations. After 6 weeks, a removable splint is provided and a gradual, progressive, active range of motion program is begun.

Galeazzi Fracture

A Galeazzi fracture represents a diaphyseal fracture of the radius with an associated DRUJ dislocation. This fracture pattern is named after Riccardo Galeazzi, who in 1934 published a series of 18 patients with this fracture pattern.[45] The Galeazzi fracture occurs at least 4 to 5 cm proximal to the radiocarpal joint.[46] The mechanism is typically high-energy trauma, such as a motor vehicle accident or a fall from a height.[47,48] The pathomechanics of the injury is thought to be wrist hyperextension with pronation.[49] Clinically and radiographically there is typically an angular deformity of the radius with radial shortening and dorsal prominence of the ulnar head (**Fig. 2**).[47]

The Galeazzi fracture is "the fracture of necessity," implying that operative fixation is required for adequate return of function.[50] Historically, nonoperative management has been associated with poor results.[49,51,52] Casting alone is associated with a poor outcome because of the strong deforming forces acting on the distal fragment, which include the pronator quadratus, brachioradialis, and thumb extensors and abductors.

Not all diaphyseal radius fractures result in an injury to the DRUJ, but it has been suggested that a quarter of all radial shaft fractures have some associated injury to the DRUJ.[53] The distance that the fracture lies from the articular surface can help the surgeon predict the likelihood of DRUJ injury. Fractures occurring within 7.5 cm from the midarticular surface of the radius have been found to have a higher incidence of concomitant DRUJ injury.[48] An associated fracture at the base of the ulnar styloid, widening of the DRUJ

on AP radiographs, dislocation of the ulna on lateral view, and greater than 5 mm of radial shortening are all suggestive of a DRUJ injury.[47,54] Plain radiographs may not always represent the true extent of soft tissue injury. Mikic[49] reported, in his study of 125 Galeazzi fractures, that while 80% of patients presented with a complete dislocation of the DRUJ, 20% presented with only radiographic evidence of subluxation, complicating the diagnosis. Clinical assessment of DRUJ should be performed intraoperatively after skeletal fixation of the radius shaft fracture. Arthroscopy has not been described as an adjunct for evaluation and treatment with Galeazzi fractures; however, as in the case of distal radius fractures, arthroscopy may prove useful for evaluation and treatment of TFCC injuries after operative repair.

A distinction has been made between simple and complex dislocations. Simple dislocations are those without interposing soft tissue in the dislocated DRUJ. Complex dislocations are those with interposing soft tissue that blocks closed reduction.[6,35,55–57] Complex dislocations are typically high-energy injuries and, to the authors' knowledge, have not been reported except in association with a fracture, especially a Galeazzi-type fracture. The most common interposing structure is the ECU tendon,[6,55–59] although other interposed structures have been described, including the extensor digiti minimi and extensor digitorum communis tendons.[56] The diagnosis of a complex dislocation is suggested by the failure of closed reduction of the DRUJ after open reduction and internal fixation (ORIF) of the radius fracture. In this situation, the interposing soft tissue blocks the closed reduction and a mushy sensation can be appreciated when reduction is attempted.[6] In this case, one must be careful not to force reduction because a radiographic reduction may be apparent even with the soft tissue interposed. In a complex dislocation, an open reduction is indicated with extraction and reduction of the soft tissue and open repair of the TFCC.[6]

Surgical approach

Galeazzi fractures are approached through a modified Henry incision within the forearm. Volar placement of the plate is performed using standard techniques. Dynamic compression plates are the authors' preferred treatment choice and have been shown to produce excellent results.[54] Screw purchase should include 6 cortices above and below the fracture site with a 3.5-mm plate (see **Fig. 2**C, D). Once the radius is reduced and fixed, the DRUJ is assessed for stability. Often a concomitant basilar ulnar styloid fracture is

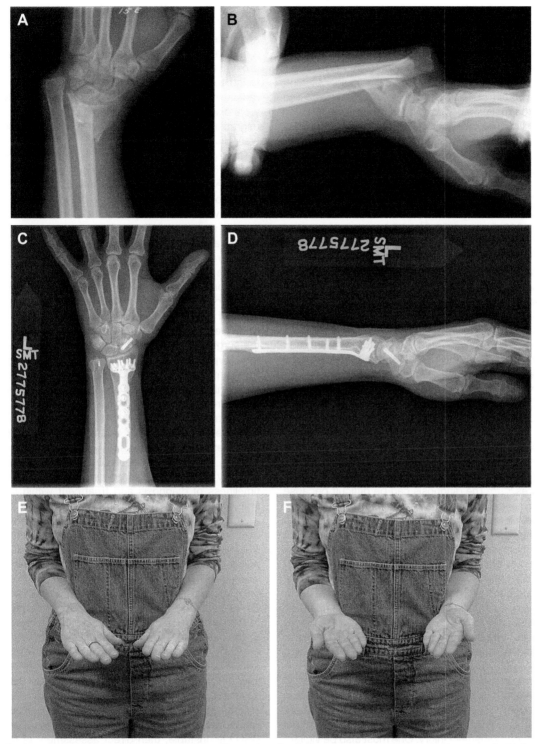

Fig. 2. Anteroposterior (*A*) and lateral (*B*) radiographs of a Galeazzi fracture with an associated scaphoid fracture. The radius fracture was treated with a long volar plate, and the TFCC was repaired with a suture anchor at the foveal insertion; radiograph 4 years after surgery shows good healing (*C, D*). Nine months after the surgery the patient regained painless forearm rotation (*E, F*).

present, which may be fixed with the tension banding technique. Persistent DRUJ instability after radial shaft fixation and ulnar styloid fixation may be addressed with arthroscopy to fully evaluate the TFCC. Significant instability may require open ligamentous repair and/or radioulnar pinning to obtain stability as previously discussed. The forearm is immobilized in a neutral position in a Munster-type cast for 4 to 6 weeks after surgery. When there is significant ulnar instability, immobilization in the more supinated position has been recommended.[60,61]

Essex-Lopresti Injury

In 1946, Curr and Coe[62] published a case report of a patient with a fracture dislocation of the radial head in combination with a dorsal dislocation of the DRUJ. In 1951, Essex-Lopresti[63] described 2 cases of a dislocation injury of the DRUJ in combination with a comminuted radial head fracture, the injury that now bears his name. The injury pattern is a manifestation of an axial compression force that results in longitudinal radioulnar disruption and involves the DRUJ, IOM, and PRUJ or radial head. The radial head is the primary constraint to proximal migration of the radius. The secondary constraints include the IOM and TFCC. In Essex-Lopresti injuries, there is loss of primary and secondary constraints. As such, the radius is freed of its constraints to the ulna and migrates proximally. These injuries can also occur in conjunction with distal radius fractures or radial shaft fractures.[64–66] The diagnosis can be difficult because the tendency is to focus on the obvious injury at the elbow.[67] The long-term problem lies in the longitudinal axial instability, which can present early or delayed as occurs after radial head excision or gradual failure of the IOM after the loss of radial head restraint. The manifestation is proximal migration of the radius, with radiocapitellar impingement proximally and ulnar impaction distally.[68,69]

The primary contributor to longitudinal forearm stability is the radial head, with the TFCC and IOM functioning as secondary stabilizers. A complete discussion of radial head fractures is beyond the scope of this article. However, the elbow must be assessed for stability and to rule out concomitant coronoid fracture and medial collateral ligament injury. One must also be vigilant in examination for axial injuries to the forearm, which would include the IOM and DRUJ. The patient typically has a history of a high-energy axial force to the hand or forearm. Examination frequently demonstrates a dorsally prominent ulna, limited wrist extension, and limited forearm rotation. Examination should include an assessment of longitudinal forearm stability.[70,71] Smith and colleagues[71] described the radius pull test in a cadaver study, whereby the radius is distracted proximally with a load of 9.1 kg. The investigators found that there was at least 3 mm of proximal radius migration when the radial head and IOM were disrupted and greater than 6 mm of proximal migration when the radial head, IOM, and TFCC were disrupted.

Radiographic evaluation includes 2 views of the elbow, forearm, and wrist. Grip views can be helpful in the assessment of dynamic radial shortening and should be compared with the contralateral normal wrist.[72] Similarly, bilateral AP wrist radiographs are obtained to evaluate differences in ulnar variance.[73] Magnetic resonance imaging and ultrasonography are important adjuncts to evaluate the soft tissue injury of the IOM.[74,75]

The primary goal of treatment is reestablishing the radiocapitellar articulation by repair or replacement of the radial head. Edwards and Jupiter[64] described a classification system that determines the surgical management of the radial head fracture. Type I fractures are those that have large fragments amenable to ORIF. Type II fractures are comminuted and ORIF is not an option. These injuries require radial head excision and prosthetic replacement. Type III injuries are chronic injuries with irreducible proximal radial head migration. The investigators recommend radial head replacement in conjunction with an ulnar shortening osteotomy procedure. Outcomes correlate to the timeliness of diagnosis and treatment within the first week.[65] Trousdale and colleagues,[65] in a summary of reported cases including their own, reported that 9 of 10 patients treated within 1 week had a satisfactory result as opposed to only 4 of 14 patients achieving a satisfactory result when treated more than 1 week after injury. Excision of the radial head is contraindicated in Essex-Lopresti injuries because there is nothing to stop proximal migration of the radius in this situation. Therefore, radial head replacement is indicated.[63,76,77] If nothing else, in this situation, the radial head replacement may function as an internal splint while the IOM, TFCC, and surrounding soft tissues are allowed to heal.

Once the radiocapitellar articulation is reestablished, the DRUJ is assessed for stability. If the DRUJ is unstable, then direct assessment of the TFCC can be performed arthroscopically. If significant instability is present or complete foveal disruption of the TFCC is noted on arthroscopy, the authors prefer direct repair of the foveal insertion with suture anchors or heavy suture through bone tunnels with or without radioulnar pinning.

The forearm is maintained in a Munster-type splint or cast until 6 weeks, when a gradual and progressive range of motion program is initiated.

Distal Radius Fractures and the DRUJ

Recent prospective studies have shown that concomitant injury to the TFCC at the time of distal radius fracture may be as high as 60% to 84%.[78,79] Despite this observation, there is still no accepted algorithm for the evaluation and treatment of these injuries.[1] The association between DRUJ injuries and distal radius fractures has been noted as early as 1814, when Abraham Colles stated, "If the surgeon proceeds to investigate the nature of this injury, he will find that the end of the ulna admits of being readily moved backward and forward."[80] Studies that used arthrography to examine TFCC injuries associated with distal radius fractures have noted an incidence of 45% to 65%.[81,82]

More recent studies using arthroscopy have revealed similar findings. Geissler and colleagues[78] examined 60 consecutive patients who had failed closed reduction and had greater than 2 mm of articular stepoff within the radius. In this study, 26 of the 60 patients were found to have an injury to the TFCC (43%); of these injuries 13 were peripheral ulnar-sided tears (Palmer 1B), 7 were radial-sided tears (Palmer 1D), and 6 were central perforations (Palmer 1A).

Lindau and colleagues[83] reported on a prospective series of 51 young patients with displaced distal radius fractures. Diagnostic nontherapeutic arthroscopy was performed on all patients. The investigators found that 43 patients (84%) had an injury of the TFCC. Worse outcomes were associated with DRUJ instability. At a median follow-up of 12 months, 19 patients (37%) had DRUJ instability, including 10 of the 11 patients diagnosed with complete avulsion at the time of arthroscopy and 7 of the 32 patients with partial peripheral or central tears.[83] Based on these studies, one can conclude that TFCC injury is commonly associated with distal radius fractures and if untreated may increase long-term morbidity.

Diagnosis of DRUJ instability after distal radius fracture

Diagnosis of DRUJ instability based on physical examination is difficult after distal radius fracture injury in the nonanesthetized patient. Therefore, stability is best assessed intraoperatively after fracture fixation in an anesthetized patient. A certain amount of laxity may be normal, and therefore comparison with the contralateral side may be necessary. Lindau and colleagues[83] reported the sensitivity and specificity of clinical diagnosis of

0.59 and 0.96, respectively. It has been suggested that if greater than 1 cm of dorsal-to-palmar translation is present, instability should be assumed.[84]

Prereduction radiographic findings may help to increase the surgeon's suspicion of DRUJ injury. Cadaveric studies suggest that if there is no evidence for an ulnar styloid fracture but the preoperative radiographs reveal significant shortening of the radius relative to the ulna (>7 mm), then a disruption of the DRUJ ligaments has likely occurred.[85] Four additional signs that may indicate DRUJ injury include (1) ulnar styloid base fracture, (2) widening of the DRUJ interval on AP radiographs, (3) dislocation of the DRUJ on lateral radiographs, and (4) more than 5 mm of radial shortening.[54] May and colleagues[86] noted a correlation with distal radius comminution and DRUJ instability; however, other studies have not shown a clear correlation between radiographic findings and DRUJ instability.[60,78,79,83,87] In Lindau and colleagues'[83] prospective study of 51 patients, the investigators found no correlation between radiographic findings (at the time of injury or at follow-up) and DRUJ instability.

A CT scan can provide additional information and may be obtained in the acute setting to further study distal radius fractures. Axial views of the DRUJ can be compared with the contralateral side. Subluxation or frank dislocation may often be identified in addition to bony fragments suggestive of palmar or radioulnar joint ligamentous avulsions (Fig. 3).[39,88]

If radiographs are nondiagnostic and the physical examination is suggestive of instability after

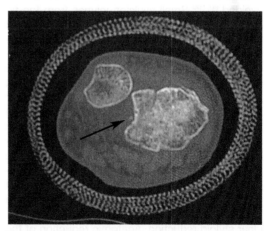

Fig. 3. Axial CT scan of a dorsal dislocation with distal radius fracture involving the sigmoid notch. The small osteochondral fragment (*arrow*) was found at surgery to represent the palmar radioulnar ligament. (*From* Carlsen B, Rizzo M, Moran S. Soft-tissue injuries associated with distal radius fractures. Operat Tech Orthop 2009;19(2):107–18; with permission.)

fracture reduction, the authors prefer arthroscopy of the TFCC to evaluate for injury. This approach allows for the possibility of immediate open repair with suture anchors or heavy suture through bone tunnels with or without radioulnar pinning.

Management of ulnar styloid fractures

Frykman[89] included fractures of the ulnar styloid in his classification system for distal radius fractures. He believed that concomitant fractures of the ulnar styloid were predictive of worse outcomes. Several clinical studies have supported this claim.[90–92] Oskarsson and colleagues[91] found ulnar styloid fractures to be associated with a greater loss of mobility and postoperative grip strength when comparing outcomes in patients with distal radius fractures. In addition, Stoffelen and colleagues,[92] in a prospective study of 272 patients, found that all patients presenting with DRUJ instability after distal radius fracture had suffered an ulnar styloid fracture at the time of the original injury. Knirk and Jupiter[90] found, in their long-term outcome study of patients with distal radius fractures, that ulnar styloid nonunions were associated with poorer outcomes. Conversely, other authors have noted no clear association between ulnar styloid fractures and overall outcomes.[93–98] Furthermore, studies using arthroscopy have suggested that an ulnar styloid fracture is not necessarily predictive of TFCC injury.[83,99]

Although the direct correlation between ulnar styloid injury and DRUJ instability is not clearly established, it does seem from the literature that ulnar styloid nonunion and malunion should be avoided.[90,100] Small avulsion injuries from the tip of the styloid are likely to be the result of direct trauma and are unlikely to involve the fovea insertion of the TFCC; however, large fragments, especially those displaced greater than 2 mm, are more likely to be associated with disruption of the foveal insertion of the TFCC and should be fixed.[27,86,101] Ruch and colleagues[84] advocate evaluation of the ulnar styloid with a true lateral radiograph. If the ulnar styloid lies palmar to the axis of the ulnar shaft, one should suspect that the stability of the DRUJ is compromised. Thus the authors recommend repairing all large ulnar styloid fragments, if possible. The authors have found wire reduction alone or tension banding to be most effective for ulnar styloid reduction. Anatomic reduction of the ulnar styloid is usually simple if the radius has been reduced to normal anatomic alignment, especially in terms of rotation and translation of the distal radial fragments.

Large ulnar styloid fractures may be fixed through a 2- to 3-cm incision made at the ulnar aspect of the wrist, directly over the styloid. This incision may be incorporated into the 6U arthroscopic portal, if this has been used to evaluate the radius during fracture fixation. The dorsal ulnar sensory nerve can be identified running with the basilic vein and is gently retracted before opening the joint capsule. The location of the nerve may be marked on the patient before surgical intervention by understanding that its course represents a perpendicular bisection of a line connecting the ulnar styloid to the pisiform. A 0.054- or 0.062-in K wire is used to create 2 transverse drill holes above and below the fracture line within the bone. A 25- or 24-gauge steel wire may then be passed through the drill holes. The styloid fracture is then pinned using two 0.045-in K wires, and the wire is then tensioned appropriately. If the distal styloid fragment is too small for the wire to pass intraosseously, the wire is held distally beneath the K wires, which are cut short and embedded within the distal fragment. Engagement of the ulnar styloid with the K wire is aided with the use of a 14-gauge needle, which is used as a soft tissue protector during K-wire placement. Alternatively, the wire driver can be used on oscillation to protect the soft tissue. The hollow needle is used to engage the periosteum of the ulnar styloid and aids in directing the K wire. K wires may be cut and imbedded into the ulnar styloid or brought out through the skin for removal in 4 to 6 weeks. Once the styloid is repaired, the stability of the DRUJ is reassessed. If the DRUJ remains unstable, repair of the foveal attachment of the TFCC may be necessary. Often the original radiograph shows a separate bony avulsion fragment adjacent to the styloid fracture, representing the foveal insertion of the TFCC,[102,103] which may be repaired arthroscopically or through an open approach.

Sigmoid notch and dorsal ulnar and volar ulnar corner fractures

Distal radius fractures often present with some injury to the lunate facet, more commonly the dorsal ulnar corner, and may also include the volar ulnar corner (marginal) fragment (which can also present with radiocarpal subluxation). These fractures may present with an unstable DRUJ because they include either the dorsal or the volar origin of the radioulnar ligaments. When these fracture fragments are present, if instability is present after reduction and fixation of the radius fracture, then further attention is directed to ensure the reduction and stability of these fragments. Preoperative CT scanning is extremely helpful in identifying these difficult fracture patterns when they are suspected on plain radiographs.

With current locking volar plating systems used to treat distal radius fractures, many of these larger dorsal ulnar fragments can be reduced and then captured by the pegs or screws through the volar plate. However, smaller or more ulnar, dorsal, and distal fragments may not be able to be stabilized without dorsal exposure, reduction, and fragment-specific fixation. On rare occasions, the sigmoid notch may be unstable with a shearing-type subchondral injury (**Fig. 4**). Reduction of these fractures can often be achieved without a dorsal incision, but closed reduction of the dorsal fragment is helped considerably by near anatomic reduction of the radial length, volar tilt, radial inclination, and radiocarpal articular surface. When trying to capture these smaller fragments, close to the DRUJ, one must be careful to make certain that no pins, screws, or pegs are placed within the DRUJ or the lunate facet. When the reduction or fixation is not obtainable without an incision, the dorsal fractures may be approached through the floor of the fourth extensor compartment. This exposure can also allow for DRUJ arthrotomy, through the floor of the fifth extensor compartment, to assist with reduction of the sigmoid notch if needed. The fragment can then be stabilized with K wires, a small plate, or fragment-specific fixation or with the distal and ulnar screws from the volar plate. Dorsal plates should always be applied with careful attention to minimize any prominence and may need to be removed if any tendon irritation is noticed. If there is any concern that the fracture requires specific protection, then the forearm is immobilized for

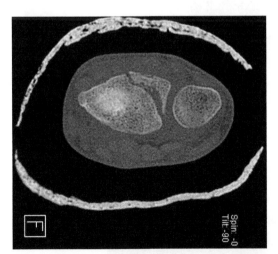

Fig. 4. Axial CT scan of a shear-type injury to the sigmoid notch. The fragment includes the radial attachment of the dorsal radioulnar ligament with a small amount of subchondral bone and dorsal comminution.

the first few weeks in a Munster-type splint in neutral forearm rotation. Early gentle 30° pronation or 30° supination forearm rotation at 2 to 3 weeks with a removable Munster splint provides a good balance of protection and motion.

Although the flexor carpi radialis approach is the most common for volar plating, the volar marginal fragment may be approached using a window on the ulnar side of the flexor tendons and radial side of the flexi carpi ulnaris (FCU) and ulnar nerve and artery. Again careful reduction and fixation is completed using either figure-of-eight suture, tension band, or fragment-specific fixation as needed.[104] Careful physical and fluoroscopic examination should be conducted to confirm the reduction and stability of the fracture fragments and the DRUJ.

Distal Ulna Fractures

Lafontaine and colleagues[105] have described the potential instability of combined distal radius and ulna fractures, particularly in patients older than 60 years. Although conservative treatment of distal ulna fractures typically is not related to late instability of the DRUJ, complications have been reported within a series of 19 (6%) distal ulna fractures that accompanied 320 distal radius fractures. Complications included 2 comminuted distal ulna fractures that were associated with nonunion, 4 of 5 simple neck fractures that had marked restriction of rotation, and 3 other cases that had fracture callus encroachment of the DRUJ that limited forearm rotation.[106] McKee and colleagues,[107] Ring and colleagues,[108] and Fernandez and colleagues[109] have reported on the potential complications, especially nonunion of the radius, with combined distal radius and distal ulna fractures.

In the authors' experience with newer locked volar plating techniques that stabilize the distal radius, many distal ulna fractures are relatively stable after reduction and stabilization of the distal radius fracture and may be treated with supplemental immobilization in a Munster-type splint or cast in neutral forearm rotation.[110] However, unstable, comminuted, or displaced distal ulnar neck and head fractures that accompany distal radius fractures may benefit from surgical treatment.[110,111] With current techniques available to stabilize distal ulna fractures, an attempt at reduction and fixation, when required, is important to maintain the most normal DRUJ congruence, stability, and motion. Options for operative fixation of these fractures include percutaneous K wires, which provide support, even with osteoporotic bone, but this technique requires postoperative immobilization and has morbidity associated with pin site irritation and infection. ORIF may allow secure fixation and earlier motion, but internal fixation may also be challenging because of small, comminuted, or osteoporotic fracture fragments. Plate position on the ulna requires careful attention so that it does not interfere with the DRUJ. The subcutaneous location of the bone and the location of the superficial branch of the ulnar nerve also emphasize the importance of a relatively low-profile implant to minimize symptoms from prominent hardware. When considering ORIF of the distal ulna (head and neck), smaller plate sizes may be appropriate, but traditional plate sizes should be maintained when stabilizing more diaphyseal or metadiaphyseal ulna fractures.

Good results have been reported after ORIF of distal ulna fractures that were associated with distal radius fractures with either condylar blade plate fixation[111] or 2-mm locking plate fixation (**Fig. 5**).[110] Results were favorable in each series with respect to union, motion, and function. The condylar ulnar plate was removed in 7 of 24 patients, and no locking plates required removal; this difference may have been related more to surgeon preference toward plate removal.[110,111]

Locking plate fixation offers a few potential advantages over condylar blade plate fixation. Locking plates allow for a lag-type locking screw and also for more than 1 locked peg to be inserted into the distal fragment, which may enhance articular reduction and stability. In either case, a low profile plate is advantageous when trying to minimize hardware prominence in this subcutaneous location. Stable fixation of the ulnar head fracture

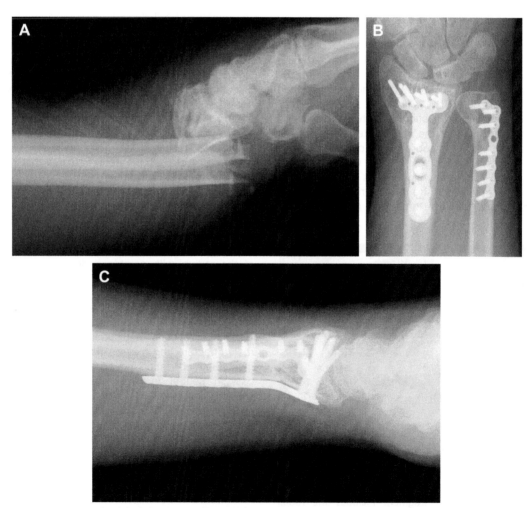

Fig. 5. Comminuted, displaced distal radius fracture and distal ulna fracture (A) fixed with a 2.0-mm locking plate of the distal ulna fracture and volar locking plate fixation of the distal radius fracture as shown on AP (B) and lateral (C) views.

allows for early motion of the DRUJ and ideally may help preserve forearm rotation.

These fractures are typically approached from the ulnar aspect of the wrist, in the ECU-FCU interval, and require careful identification and protection of the dorsal sensory branch of the ulnar nerve. In general, the most helpful step in obtaining a reduced ulna is a well-aligned distal radius and a reduced DRUJ. All efforts should be made to obtain an anatomic reduction and secure fixation of the distal radius, especially with respect to length and correction of the coronal plane translation, in addition to the volar tilt and radial inclination. The distal ulna fracture can then be reduced and temporarily stabilized with any technique, and K wires are often helpful to hold the initial reduction. Definitive fixation can then often be achieved through fragment-specific, fixed-angle, or locked-plate fixation. In addition, if there is an associated ulnar styloid fracture or foveal avulsion, these may be incorporated into the repair. In general, if the comminuted, intraarticular, or displaced distal ulna fracture can be repaired, especially in younger patients, it is likely preferable to either resection or implant arthroplasty.

SUMMARY

Acute dislocations of the DRUJ can occur in isolation or in association with a fracture to the distal radius, radial metadiaphysis (Galeazzi fracture), or radial head (Essex-Lopresti injury). Distal ulna fractures may occur in isolation or in combination with a distal radius fracture. Both injury patterns are associated with relatively high energy. Successful outcomes are predicated on anatomic restoration and stability of the DRUJ.

REFERENCES

1. Carlsen B, Rizzo M, Moran S. Soft-tissue injuries associated with distal radius fractures. Operat Tech Orthop 2009;19(2):107–18.
2. af Ekenstam FW, Palmer AK, Glisson RR. The load on the radius and ulna in different positions of the wrist and forearm. A cadaver study. Acta Orthop Scand 1984;55(3):363–5.
3. Drobner WS, Hausman MR. The distal radioulnar joint. Hand Clin 1992;8(4):631–44.
4. Epner RA, Bowers WH, Guilford WB. Ulnar variance—the effect of wrist positioning and roentgen filming technique. J Hand Surg Am 1982;7(3):298–305.
5. Palmer AK, Werner FW. Biomechanics of the distal radioulnar joint. Clin Orthop Relat Res 1984;187:26–35.
6. Bruckner JD, Lichtman DM, Alexander AH. Complex dislocations of the distal radioulnar joint. Recognition and management. Clin Orthop Relat Res 1992;275:90–103.
7. Linscheid RL. Biomechanics of the distal radioulnar joint. Clin Orthop Relat Res 1992;275:46–55.
8. Ray RD, Johnson RJ, Jameson RM. Rotation of the forearm; an experimental study of pronation and supination. J Bone Joint Surg Am 1951;33(4):993–6.
9. Stuart PR, Berger RA, Linscheid RL, et al. The dorsopalmar stability of the distal radioulnar joint. J Hand Surg Am 2000;25(4):689–99.
10. Tolat AR, Stanley JK, Trail IA. A cadaveric study of the anatomy and stability of the distal radioulnar joint in the coronal and transverse planes. J Hand Surg Br 1996;21(5):587–94.
11. Palmer AK, Werner FW. The triangular fibrocartilage complex of the wrist—anatomy and function. J Hand Surg Am 1981;6(2):153–62.
12. Bednar MS, Arnoczky SP, Weiland AJ. The microvasculature of the triangular fibrocartilage complex: its clinical significance. J Hand Surg Am 1991;16(6):1101–5.
13. Hagert CG. Distal radius fracture and the distal radioulnar joint—anatomical considerations. Handchir Mikrochir Plast Chir 1994;26(1):22–6.
14. af Ekenstam F. Anatomy of the distal radioulnar joint. Clin Orthop Relat Res 1992;275:14–8.
15. Schuind F, An KN, Berglund L, et al. The distal radioulnar ligaments: a biomechanical study. J Hand Surg Am 1991;16(6):1106–14.
16. Kihara H, Short WH, Werner FW, et al. The stabilizing mechanism of the distal radioulnar joint during pronation and supination. J Hand Surg Am 1995;20(6):930–6.
17. Kleinman WB. Stability of the distal radioulna joint: biomechanics, pathophysiology, physical diagnosis, and restoration of function what we have learned in 25 years. J Hand Surg Am 2007;32(7):1086–106.
18. Xu J, Tang JB. In vivo changes in lengths of the ligaments stabilizing the distal radioulnar joint. J Hand Surg Am 2009;34(1):40–5.
19. Rose-Innes AP. Anterior dislocation of the ulna at the inferior radio-ulnar joint. Case report, with a discussion of the anatomy of rotation of the forearm. J Bone Joint Surg Br 1960;42:515–21.
20. Buterbaugh GA, Palmer AK. Fractures and dislocations of the distal radioulnar joint. Hand Clin 1988;4(3):361–75.
21. Hui FC, Linscheid RL. Ulnotriquetral augmentation tenodesis: a reconstructive procedure for dorsal subluxation of the distal radioulnar joint. J Hand Surg Am 1982;7(3):230–6.
22. Moritomo H, Noda K, Goto A, et al. Interosseous membrane of the forearm: length change of

ligaments during forearm rotation. J Hand Surg Am 2009;34(4):685–91.

23. Noda K, Goto A, Murase T, et al. Interosseous membrane of the forearm: an anatomical study of ligament attachment locations. J Hand Surg Am 2009;34(3):415–22.

24. Watanabe H, Berger RA, Berglund LJ, et al. Contribution of the interosseous membrane to distal radioulnar joint constraint. J Hand Surg Am 2005; 30(6):1164–71.

25. Skahen JR 3rd, Palmer AK, Werner FW, et al. The interosseous membrane of the forearm: anatomy and function. J Hand Surg Am 1997;22(6):981–5.

26. Hotchkiss RN, An KN, Sowa DT, et al. An anatomic and mechanical study of the interosseous membrane of the forearm: pathomechanics of proximal migration of the radius. J Hand Surg Am 1989;14(2 Pt 1):256–61.

27. Mikic ZD. Treatment of acute injuries of the triangular fibrocartilage complex associated with distal radioulnar joint instability. J Hand Surg Am 1995; 20(2):319–23.

28. Desault. Cadaver case; typical luxation; no history. J de Chirurgie 1777;i(I):78.

29. Cotton FJ, Brickley WJ. Luxation of the ulna forward at the wrist (without fracture): with report of a case. Ann Surg 1912;55(3):368–74.

30. Albert MJ, Engber WD. Dorsal dislocation of the distal radioulnar joint secondary to plastic deformation of the ulna. J Orthop Trauma 1990;4(4):466–9.

31. Dameron TB Jr. Traumatic dislocation of the distal radio-ulnar joint. Clin Orthop Relat Res 1972;83: 55–63.

32. Heiple KG, Freehafer AA, Van'T Hof A. Isolated traumatic dislocation of the distal end of the ulna or distal radio-ulnar joint. J Bone Joint Surg Am 1962;44:1387–94.

33. Morrissy RT, Nalebuff EA. Dislocation of the distal radioulnar joint: anatomy and clues to prompt diagnosis. Clin Orthop Relat Res 1979;144:154–8.

34. Alexander AH. Bilateral traumatic dislocation of the distal radioulnar joint, ulna dorsal: case report and review of the literature. Clin Orthop Relat Res 1977; 129:238–44.

35. Hanel DP, Scheid DK. Irreducible fracture-dislocation of the distal radioulnar joint secondary to entrapment of the extensor carpi ulnaris tendon. Clin Orthop Relat Res 1988;234:56–60.

36. Bruckner JD, Alexander AH, Lichtman DM. Acute dislocations of the distal radioulnar joint. Instr Course Lect 1996;45:27–36.

37. Milch H. So-called dislocation of the lower end of the ulna. Ann Surg 1942;116(2):282–92.

38. Hagert CG. The distal radioulnar joint. Hand Clin 1987;3(1):41–50.

39. Mino DE, Palmer AK, Levinsohn EM. The role of radiography and computerized tomography in the

diagnosis of subluxation and dislocation of the distal radioulnar joint. J Hand Surg Am 1983;8(1): 23–31.

40. Yang Z, Mann FA, Gilula LA, et al. Scaphopisocapitate alignment: criterion to establish a neutral lateral view of the wrist. Radiology 1997;205(3):865–9.

41. Mino DE, Palmer AK, Levinsohn EM. Radiography and computerized tomography in the diagnosis of incongruity of the distal radio-ulnar joint. A prospective study. J Bone Joint Surg Am 1985; 67(2):247–52.

42. Park MJ, Kim JP. Reliability and normal values of various computed tomography methods for quantifying distal radioulnar joint translation. J Bone Joint Surg Am 2008;90(1):145–53.

43. Garrigues GE, Aldridge JM 3rd. Acute irreducible distal radioulnar joint dislocation. A case report. J Bone Joint Surg Am 2007;89(7):1594–7.

44. Ruch DS, Lumsden BC, Papadonikolakis A. Distal radius fractures: a comparison of tension band wiring versus ulnar outrigger external fixation for the management of distal radioulnar instability. J Hand Surg Am 2005;30(5):969–77.

45. Galeazzi R. Uber ein besonderes Syndrom bei Verlrtzunger in Bereick der Unter Armknochen. Arch Orthop Unfallchir 1934;35:557–62 [in German].

46. Faierman E, Jupiter JB. The management of acute fractures involving the distal radio-ulnar joint and distal ulna. Hand Clin 1998;14:213–29.

47. Giannoulis FS, Sotereanos DG. Galeazzi fractures and dislocations. Hand Clin 2007;23(2):153–63, v.

48. Rettig ME, Raskin KB. Galeazzi fracture-dislocation: a new treatment-oriented classification. J Hand Surg Am 2001;26(2):228–35.

49. Mikic ZD. Galeazzi fracture-dislocations. J Bone Joint Surg Am 1975;57:1071–80.

50. Anderson LD, Meyer FN. Fractures of the shafts of the radius and ulna. In: Rockwood CA, Green DP, editors. Fractures in adults. Philadelphia: JB Lippincott Co; 1991. p. 728.

51. Hughston JC. Fracture of the distal radial shaft. Mistakes in management. J Bone Joint Surg Am 1957;39:249–64.

52. Reckling FW. Unstable fracture-dislocations of the forearm (Montaggia and Galeazzi lesions). J Bone Joint Surg Am 1982;64:857–63.

53. Ring D, Rhim R, Carpenter C, et al. Isolated radial shaft fractures are more common than Galeazzi fractures. J Hand Surg Am 2006;31(1):17–21.

54. Moore TM, Klein JP, Patzakis MJ, et al. Results of compression-plating of closed Galeazzi fractures. J Bone Joint Surg Am 1985;67(7):1015–21.

55. Cetti NE. An unusual cause of blocked reduction of the Galeazzi injury. Injury 1977;9(1):59–61.

56. Jenkins NH, Mintowt-Czyz WJ, Fairclough JA. Irreducible dislocation of the distal radioulnar joint. Injury 1987;18(1):40–3.

57. Alexander AH, Lichtman DM. Irreducible distal radioulnar joint occurring in a Galeazzi fracture – case report. J Hand Surg Am 1981;6(3):258–61.

58. Itoh Y, Horiuchi Y, Takahashi M, et al. Extensor tendon involvement in Smith's and Galeazzi's fractures. J Hand Surg Am 1987;12(4):535–40.

59. Paley D, Rubenstein J, McMurtry RY. Irreducible dislocation of distal radial ulnar joint. Orthop Rev 1986;15(4):228–31.

60. Geissler WB, Fernandez DL, Lamey DM. Distal radioulnar joint injuries associated with fractures of the distal radius. Clin Orthop Relat Res 1996;327:135–46.

61. Ginn TA, Ruch DS, Yang CC, et al. Use of a distraction plate for distal radial fractures with metaphyseal and diaphyseal comminution. Surgical technique. J Bone Joint Surg Am 2006;88(Suppl 1 Pt 1):29–36.

62. Curr JF, Coe WA. Dislocation of the inferior radioulnar joint. Br J Surg 1946;34:74–7.

63. Essex-Lopresti P. Fractures of the radial head with distal radio-ulnar dislocation; report of two cases. J Bone Joint Surg Br 1951;33(2):244–7.

64. Edwards GS Jr, Jupiter JB. Radial head fractures with acute distal radioulnar dislocation. Essex-Lopresti revisited. Clin Orthop Relat Res 1988;234:61–9.

65. Trousdale RT, Amadio PC, Cooney WP, et al. Radioulnar dissociation. A review of twenty cases. J Bone Joint Surg Am 1992;74(10):1486–97.

66. Eglseder WA, Hay M. Combined Essex-Lopresti and radial shaft fractures: case report. J Trauma 1993;34(2):310–2.

67. Adams JE, Culp RW, Osterman AL. Interosseous membrane reconstruction for the Essex-Lopresti injury. J Hand Surg Am 2010;35(1):129–36.

68. Shepard MF, Markolf KL, Dunbar AM. The effects of partial and total interosseous membrane transection on load sharing in the cadaver forearm. J Orthop Res 2001;19(4):587–92.

69. Shepard MF, Markolf KL, Dunbar AM. Effects of radial head excision and distal radial shortening on load-sharing in cadaver forearms. J Bone Joint Surg Am 2001;83(1):92–100.

70. Davidson PA, Moseley JB Jr, Tullos HS. Radial head fracture. A potentially complex injury. Clin Orthop Relat Res 1993;297:224–30.

71. Smith AM, Urbanosky LR, Castle JA, et al. Radius pull test: predictor of longitudinal forearm instability. J Bone Joint Surg Am 2002;84(11):1970–6.

72. Swanson AB, Jaeger SH, La Rochelle D. Comminuted fractures of the radial head. The role of silicone-implant replacement arthroplasty. J Bone Joint Surg Am 1981;63(7):1039–49.

73. Marcotte AL, Osterman AL. Longitudinal radioulnar dissociation: identification and treatment of acute and chronic injuries. Hand Clin 2007;23(2):195–208, vi.

74. Starch DW, Dabezies EJ. Magnetic resonance imaging of the interosseous membrane of the forearm. J Bone Joint Surg Am 2001;83(2):235–8.

75. Wallace AL, Walsh WR, van Rooijen M, et al. The interosseous membrane in radio-ulnar dissociation. J Bone Joint Surg Br 1997;79(3):422–7.

76. Moro JK, Werier J, MacDermid JC, et al. Arthroplasty with a metal radial head for unreconstructible fractures of the radial head. J Bone Joint Surg Am 2001;83(8):1201–11.

77. Taylor TK, O'Connor BT. The effect upon the inferior radio-ulnar joint of excision of the head of the radius in adults. J Bone Joint Surg Br 1964;46:83–8.

78. Geissler WB, Freeland AE, Savoie FH, et al. Intracarpal soft-tissue lesions associated with an intraarticular fracture of the distal end of the radius. J Bone Joint Surg Am 1996;78(3):357–65.

79. Lindau T, Arner M, Hagberg L. Intraarticular lesions in distal fractures of the radius in young adults. A descriptive arthroscopic study in 50 patients. J Hand Surg Br 1997;22(5):638–43.

80. Colles A. Historical paper on the fracture of the carpal extremity of the radius (1814). Injury 1970;2(1):48–50.

81. Mohanti RC, Kar N. Study of triangular fibrocartilage of the wrist joint in Colles' fracture. Injury 1980;11(4):321–4.

82. Fontes D, Lenoble E, de Somer B, et al. [Lesions of the ligaments associated with distal fractures of the radius. 58 intraoperative arthrographies]. Ann Chir Main Memb Super 1992;11(2):119–25 [in French].

83. Lindau T, Adlercreutz C, Aspenberg P. Peripheral tears of the triangular fibrocartilage complex cause distal radioulnar joint instability after distal radial fractures. J Hand Surg Am 2000;25(3):464–8.

84. Ruch DS, Weiland AJ, Wolfe SW, et al. Current concepts in the treatment of distal radial fractures. Instr Course Lect 2004;53:389–401.

85. Adams BD. Effects of radial deformity on distal radioulnar joint mechanics. J Hand Surg Am 1993;18:492–8.

86. May MM, Lawton JN, Blazar PE. Ulnar styloid fractures associated with distal radius fractures: incidence and implications for distal radioulnar joint instability. J Hand Surg Am 2002;27(6):965–71.

87. Geissler WB. Arthroscopically assisted reduction of intra-articular fractures of the distal radius. Hand Clin 1995;11(1):19–29.

88. Chidgey LK. Treatment of acute and chronic instability of the distal radio-ulnar joint. Hand Clin 1998;14:297–303.

89. Frykman G. Fracture of the distal radius including sequelae—shoulder-hand-finger syndrome, disturbance in the distal radio-ulnar joint and impairment of nerve function. A clinical and experimental study. Acta Orthop Scand 1967;(Suppl 108):3+.

90. Knirk JL, Jupiter JB. Intra-articular fractures of the distal end of the radius in young adults. J Bone Joint Surg Am 1986;68(5):647–59.

91. Oskarsson GV, Aaser P, Hjall A. Do we underestimate the predictive value of the ulnar styloid affection in Colles fractures? Arch Orthop Trauma Surg 1997;116(6–7):341–4.

92. Stoffelen D, De Smet L, Broos P. The importance of the distal radioulnar joint in distal radial fractures. J Hand Surg Br 1998;23(4):507–11.

93. Aro HT, Koivunen T. Minor axial shortening of the radius affects outcome of Colles' fracture treatment. J Hand Surg Am 1991;16(3):392–8.

94. Villar RN, Marsh D, Rushton N, et al. Three years after Colles' fracture. A prospective review. J Bone Joint Surg Br 1987;69(4):635–8.

95. Roysam GS. The distal radio-ulnar joint in Colles' fractures. J Bone Joint Surg Br 1993;75(1):58–60.

96. Kim JK, Koh YD, Do NH. Should an ulnar styloid fracture be fixed following volar plate fixation of a distal radial fracture? J Bone Joint Surg Am 2010;92(1):1–6.

97. Sammer DM, Shah HM, Shauver MJ, et al. The effect of ulnar styloid fractures on patient-rated outcomes after volar locking plating of distal radius fractures. J Hand Surg Am 2009;34(9):1595–602.

98. Souer JS, Ring D, Matschke S, et al. Effect of an unrepaired fracture of the ulnar styloid base on outcome after plate-and-screw fixation of a distal radial fracture. J Bone Joint Surg Am 2009;91(4):830–8.

99. Richards RS, Bennett JD, Roth JH, et al. Arthroscopic diagnosis of intra-articular soft tissue injuries associated with distal radial fractures. J Hand Surg Am 1997;22(5):772–6.

100. af Ekenstam F, Jakobsson OP, Wadin K. Repair of the triangular ligament in Colles' fracture. No effect in a prospective randomized study. Acta Orthop Scand 1989;60(4):393–6.

101. Nakamura R, Horii E, Imaeda T, et al. Ulnar styloid malunion with dislocation of the distal radioulnar joint. J Hand Surg Br 1998;23(2):173–5.

102. Melone CP Jr, Nathan R. Traumatic disruption of the triangular fibrocartilage complex. Pathoanatomy. Clin Orthop Relat Res 1992;275:65–73.

103. Adams BD, Samani JE, Holley KA. Triangular fibrocartilage injury: a laboratory model. J Hand Surg Am 1996;21(2):189–93.

104. Harness NG, Jupiter JB, Orbay JL, et al. Loss of fixation of the volar lunate facet fragment in fractures of the distal part of the radius. J Bone Joint Surg Am 2004;86(9):1900–8.

105. Lafontaine M, Hardy D, Delince P. Stability assessment of distal radius fractures. Injury 1989;20(4):208–10.

106. Biyani A, Simison AJ, Klenerman L. Fractures of the distal radius and ulna. J Hand Surg Br 1995;20(3):357–64.

107. McKee MD, Waddell JP, Yoo D, et al. Nonunion of distal radial fractures associated with distal ulnar shaft fractures: a report of four cases. J Orthop Trauma 1997;11(1):49–53.

108. Ring D, Rhim R, Carpenter C, et al. Comminuted diaphyseal fractures of the radius and ulna: does bone grafting affect nonunion rate? J Trauma 2005;59(2):438–41 [discussion: 442].

109. Fernandez DL, Capo JT, Gonzalez E. Corrective osteotomy for symptomatic increased ulnar tilt of the distal end of the radius. J Hand Surg Am 2001;26(4):722–32.

110. Dennison DG. Open reduction and internal locked fixation of unstable distal ulna fractures with concomitant distal radius fracture. J Hand Surg Am 2007;32(6):801–5.

111. Ring D, McCarty LP, Campbell D, et al. Condylar blade plate fixation of unstable fractures of the distal ulna associated with fracture of the distal radius. J Hand Surg Am 2004;29(1):103–9.

The Management of Chronic Distal Radioulnar Instability

Sanjeev Kakar, MD, MRCS, MBA[a], Brian T. Carlsen, MD[b],
Steven L. Moran, MD[b], Richard A. Berger, MD, PhD[a],*

KEYWORDS

- Chronic distal radioulnar joint instability
- Soft tissue reconstruction • DRUJ ligament reconstruction
- Post-traumatic DRUJ instability

Chronic distal radioulnar joint (DRUJ) instability can result from dislocations, fractures of the radius and ulna, malunions, and ligament injuries. Other conditions presenting with ulnar-sided wrist pain can coexist or mimic these symptoms, including triangular fibrocartilage complex (TFCC) tears, extensor carpi ulnaris (ECU) subluxation and/or tendonitis, DRUJ arthritis, lunotriquetral ligament attenuation and/or tear, ulnocarpal impingement, and ulnocarpal instability. If left untreated, instability of the DRUJ leads to alterations in its normal kinematics and can result in chronic functional impairment and disability secondary to marked pain, decreased grip strength, and arthritis. The most common form of instability is when the distal ulna is displaced dorsally with respect to the radius. This type of instability is most pronounced in full pronation as opposed to volar subluxating instability, which is most noted in supination.[1]

Given the shallower dimension and greater radius of curvature of the sigmoid notch compared with the ulna head, there is a degree of dorsal/palmar translation during forearm rotation.[1,2] This architecture, however, can lend itself toward inherent DRUJ instability. Stuart and colleagues[3] demonstrated that only 20% of dorsopalmar stability is caused by bony constraints. However, this can vary, given the variations of the sigmoid notch in the transverse plane. Tolat and colleagues[4] performed a cadaveric study classifying the different types of sigmoid notch

morphologies and reported that 42% of wrists had a flat face, whereas the remainder were a combination of C types, S types, and ski slopes. In 98% of the specimens, an osteocartilaginous volar lip was noted, thereby providing additional restraint to palmar dislocation of the ulna (**Fig. 1**). In a cadaveric study by af Ekenstam and Hagert,[5] the radius of curvature of the sigmoid notch was found to be approximately 50% greater than the ulna head, permitting rotation and sliding during pronation and supination. Indeed, in maximal supination, the articular contact area consists of only 2 to 3 mm at the palmar lip.

Therefore, stability is predominantly provided by the encompassing soft tissue sleeve, which is divided into dynamic and static stabilizers. The former include the ECU and pronator quadratus, whereas the latter are composed of the DRUJ capsule, ulnotriquetral and ulnolunate ligaments, interosseous membrane, and TFCC (**Fig. 2**). In terms of the static stabilizers, the primary stabilizers of the DRUJ are the palmar and dorsal radioulnar ligaments. These stabilizers originate from the distal margins of the DRUJ and appear as thickenings at the junction of the TFCC, DRUJ, and ulnocarpal capsule. The cartilaginous disk is located centrally between these ligaments. As the radioulnar ligaments pass toward the ulna, they divide into a superficial limb, which inserts into the ulnar styloid, and a deep limb that attaches to the fovea. These ligaments remain in a relaxed

[a] Division of Hand Surgery, Department of Orthopaedic Surgery, Mayo Clinic, 200 1st Street SW, Rochester, MN 55905, USA
[b] Division of Plastic Surgery, Department of Surgery, Mayo Clinic, 200 1st Street SW, Rochester, MN 55905, USA
* Corresponding author.
E-mail address: berger.richard@mayo.edu

Hand Clin 26 (2010) 517–528
doi:10.1016/j.hcl.2010.05.010
0749-0712/10/$ – see front matter © 2010 Published by Elsevier Inc.

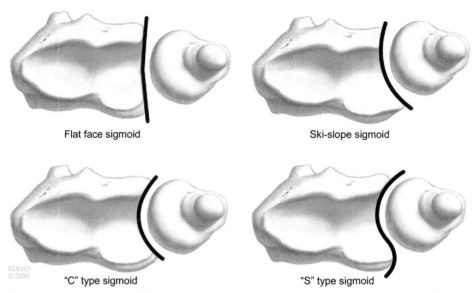

Flat face sigmoid

Ski-slope sigmoid

"C" type sigmoid

"S" type sigmoid

MAYO
© 2010

Fig. 1. The 4 anatomic variations of the sigmoid notch. (*From* Tolat AR, Stanley JK, Trail IA. A cadaveric study of the anatomy and stability of the distal radioulnar joint in the coronal and transverse planes. J Hand Surg Br 1996;21(5):592; with permission.)

position until terminal pronation and supination, thereby permitting palmar and dorsal translation of the ulna head over several millimeters.[6–8]

In trying to elucidate a role of the stabilizing structures during wrist motion, Kihara and colleagues[6] sequentially divided the dorsal and palmar radioulnar ligaments, the pronator quadratus, and the interosseous membrane. Results showed that the division of any 2 of the 4 structures did not produce DRUJ instability, whereas when all 4 were sectioned, dislocation and diastasis ensued. When the interosseous membrane was disrupted, the dorsal radioulnar ligament was taut in pronation, with the palmar ligament being the most important restraint to dislocation in supination. Similar results have been reported by other investigators.[7] In apparent contradistinction to these findings, af Ekenstam and Hagert[5] demonstrated that the palmar radioulnar ligament was tight in pronation; the dorsal ligament, in supination. In a cadaveric study, Stuart and coworkers[3] further examined the role of soft tissue stabilizers in dorsal/palmar stability of the DRUJ. The palmar radioulnar ligament provided the greatest restraint to dorsal ulna translocation, and a combination of the interosseous membrane and dorsal and palmar ligaments was important against palmar subluxation. The ECU subsheath did not contribute to DRUJ stability. To better replicate the in vivo environment, Gofton and colleagues[9] examined the role of static stabilizers on the kinematics of the DRUJ during simulated active motion. The investigators serially sectioned

the dorsal and palmar radioulnar ligaments, dorsal and palmar capsules, ECU subsheath, ulna collateral ligament, pronator quadratus, and interosseous membrane. They found that sectioning all the soft tissues altered the DRUJ kinematics during simulated motion. When the radioulnar ligaments and TFCC were left intact, normal DRUJ motion occurred. When these structures were divided, normal kinematics could only be seen when the remaining soft tissue constraints were uninjured. With these findings, the investigators concluded that the radioulnar ligaments and TFCC are not essential for maintaining normal DRUJ kinematics as long as the remaining soft tissues are intact. Therefore, when true instability is recognized, there is likely a concomitant injury to multiple structures.

CAUSES

Chronic instability of the DRUJ results from an acute traumatic injury that is unrecognized at the time of injury, inadequately treated, or recurrent after ineffective treatment. Acute injury to the TFCC can result from an isolated dislocation or in combination with a distal radius fracture, ulnar styloid fracture, radial shaft fracture (Galeazzi injury), or longitudinal radioulnar dissociation (Essex-Lopresti injury).

Distal radius fractures are frequently associated with ulna-sided injuries. Concerns about instability of the DRUJ in patients with an ulnar styloid fracture originate from the fact that the radioulnar

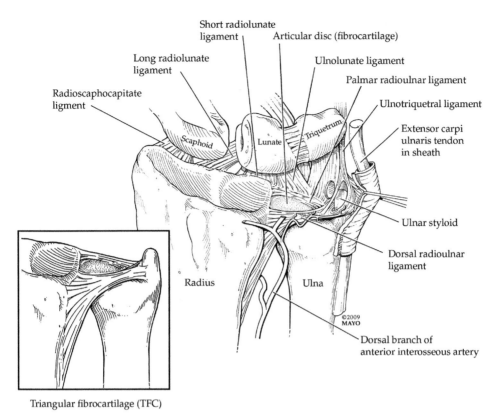

Short radiolunate ligament

Long radiolunate ligament

Radioscaphocapitate ligment

Articular disc (fibrocartilage)

Ulnolunate ligament

Palmar radioulnar ligament

Ulnotriquetral ligament

Extensor carpi ulnaris tendon in sheath

Scaphoid

Lunate

Triquetrum

Ulnar styloid

Dorsal radioulnar ligament

Radius

Ulna

©2009 MAYO

Dorsal branch of anterior interosseous artery

Triangular fibrocartilage (TFC)

TFC and Related Anatomy

Fig. 2. Primary and secondary stabilizers of the DRUJ. (*From* Carlsen B, Rizzo M, Moran S. Soft-tissue injuries associated with distal radius fractures. Operat Tech Orthop 2009;19(2):108; with permission.)

ligaments attach to the base of the styloid.[10,11] Studies have shown that there is a significant risk of TFCC injury with distal radius fracture, whether assessed using arthrography[12,13] or arthroscopy.[14] In a study by Lindau and colleagues,[15] diagnostic nontherapeutic arthroscopy was performed on young, healthy patients with distal radius fractures. Out of 51 patients, 43 had evidence of a TFCC injury. Ten of the 11 patients who had complete TFCC detachment at the time of arthroscopy had DRUJ instability at follow-up, and 7 of 32 patients diagnosed with partial peripheral or central tears had evidence of DRUJ instability at follow-up. Patients with instability had significantly worse functional outcome scores after a median follow-up of 12 months. DRUJ instability was not associated with radiographic findings at the time of injury or at follow-up examination. Ulnar styloid fracture, displacement, and nonunion did not correlate with DRUJ instability.[15]

Kim and colleagues[16] prospectively followed up 138 consecutive patients with unstable distal radius treated with open reduction and internal fixation. They reported that 76 patients had an accompanying ulnar styloid fracture (in 34 patients the bone was minimally displaced; and in 42, displaced >2 mm) that was not fixed. After an average of 19-months follow-up, the investigators did not find a significant difference between functional wrist outcomes based on grip strength, wrist range of motion, Mayo wrist score and Disabilities of the Arm, Shoulder and Hand score, and ulnar styloid fracture level or displacement. Two patients developed chronic DRUJ instability: one had an ulnar styloid fracture and the other did not. The investigators argued that it is the loss of volar tilt in healed distal radius fractures that affects DRUJ kinematics and that the presence of an ulnar styloid fracture is not significant. Therefore, although ulnar styloid fractures have previously been associated with poorer outcomes,[17–19] it is likely that anatomic reduction of the distal radius is the critical issue. The importance of anatomic reduction of the distal radius is supported by other studies.[20,21] Kihara and colleagues[21] demonstrated that more than 10° of dorsal tilt from neutral resulted in DRUJ incongruency. Pronation and supination were limited and attributed to increased tightness within the interosseous membrane. Adams[20] reported similar findings and also noted that radial shortening and decreased radial inclination adversely affected both DRUJ kinematics and distortion of the TFCC.

In addition to distal radius injuries, recognition of complex fracture dislocation patterns, such as Essex-Lopresti and Galeazzi injuries, should alert the potential of chronic DRUJ instability, if not adequately addressed. Rettig and Raskin[22] treated 40 patients who had Galeazzi fracture dislocations with open reduction and internal fixation of the radius. The investigators noted that in the 22 patients in whom the fracture was within 7.5 cm of the distal radius' articular surface, 12 were associated with intraoperative DRUJ instability. In 18 patients whose fracture was greater than 7.5 cm from the radius' articular surface, 1 patient had intraoperative DRUJ instability after open reduction and internal fixation of the radial shaft fracture.[22]

TFCC injury can also occur without osseous injury. It can be seen in patients who fall on an outstretched wrist or who have sustained a sudden rotatory injury. If left untreated, this injury can lead to chronic DRUJ instability. These patients can progress to develop mechanical symptoms at the wrist, exacerbated by activities that require forearm rotation, such as turning a screwdriver.

EVALUATION

DRUJ instability is difficult to diagnose because it can present with nonspecific signs and symptoms. Therefore, evaluation must start with a detailed history and physical examination. Patients often recount a history of a fall with the wrist in the extended and pronated position, preceding complaints of a painful clunking sensation that is exacerbated with wrist motion. This sensation is especially noticeable with twisting actions that lead to a loss of rotation secondary to pain. On examination, it is essential that the contralateral extremity be assessed because the normal range of motion and laxity of the DRUJ vary among individuals. Patients often have pain with pronation and supination of the wrist and frequently have a prominent ulna head at terminal pronation. In patients with volar instability, a slight fullness may be seen within the palmar region, with a depression noted on the dorsal wrist. Tenderness is frequently noted within the foveal region of the ulna head, which resides between the flexor carpi ulnaris tendon and ulna styloid.[23] Passive laxity should be assessed with the forearm in neutral, pronation, and supination and compared

with the uninjured side. Compression across the DRUJ may cause pain or accentuate a clunk as the ulna head dislocates and reduces within the notch. A positive result in a piano-key test is frequently noted with pain when the ulna head is depressed volarly and then released.[24] Pain may be relieved by depressing the ulna head with the thumb while simultaneously elevating the pisiform bone in patients with carpal supination and dorsal subluxation of the ulna head.[25] An additional provocative maneuver is the press test, originally described by Lester and colleagues[26] as a test with 100% sensitivity for a TFCC tear. The test was subsequently modified by Adams and Berger,[27] whereby the patients were asked to press both hands on a flat table with the forearms pronated and placed in front of them. With DRUJ instability, the ulna is more prominent dorsally and seems to sublux volar with pressure, creating a dorsal hollow.

Standard wrist radiographs should be assessed for specific signs of instability. Specifically, these include a widened DRUJ and displacement of the ulna head, either volarly or dorsally, to the radius. Radiographs should also be examined for evidence of DRUJ arthrosis and radius and ulna malunions because they have a direct effect on potential DRUJ reconstructive options (**Fig. 3**). Computed tomographic (CT) scanning provides an additional modality to evaluate for degeneration, sigmoid notch incongruity, and instability. In vivo 3-dimensional assessment of the DRUJ has been advocated as a tool to aid in detecting instability of the DRUJ.[28] Tay and colleagues[28] examined the CT scan images of 10 normal subjects whose forearms were placed through a range of maximum isometric supination to maximum isometric pronation. Results showed that during maximum isometric pronation, the ulna fovea displaced a mean of 0.51 mm dorsally and a mean of 0.13 mm volarly with maximum isometric supination. With standardized reference ranges, it may be possible to use this modality to improve detection and also quantify instabilities of the DRUJ. At the authors' institution, they include CT evaluation of both wrists in neutral, 60° pronation, and 60° supination, with neutral and stress views (pronation and supination force) at each position to assess for dynamic and static DRUJ instability.

The use of selectively placed injections of a local anesthetic can aid in the diagnosis of DRUJ instability. This is particularly useful, given the differential diagnosis of ulna-sided wrist pain that includes ulnar styloid nonunions, ECU

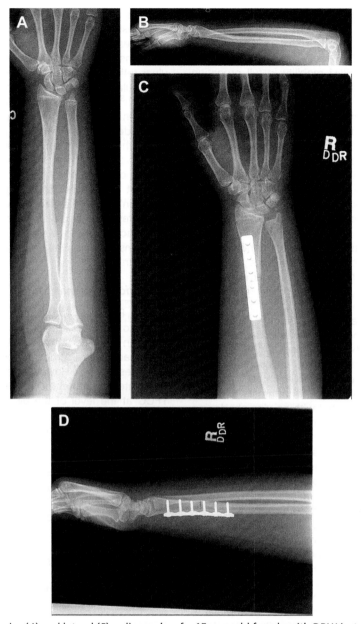

Fig. 3. Anteroposterior (*A*) and lateral (*B*) radiographs of a 15-year-old female with DRUJ instability secondary to radius malunion that required corrective radius osteotomy and fixation (*C, D*) before reconstruction of the DRUJ ligaments.

tenosynovitis versus possible subluxation, ulnocarpal abutment, lunotriquetral ligament injury, TFCC tears, dorsal ulna sensory nerve injury, and inflammatory arthropathies.

INDICATIONS AND CONTRAINDICATIONS FOR DRUJ RECONSTRUCTION

Before considering surgical reconstruction, a trial of nonoperative management is warranted because it can diminish symptoms of chronic posttraumatic DRUJ instability. In less active patients, nonoperative management can form the basis of definitive treatment, whereas in more active patients, it can serve as initial therapy to treat coexistent conditions such as ECU tendinitis. In terms of mechanism of action, functional bracing relies on hydrostatic forces to maintain the stable relationship between the radius and ulna.[29] Functional bracing was demonstrated by

Millard and colleagues[29] in a cadaveric study analyzing the effects of prefabricated commercial versus custom-made splints on DRUJ joint stability using CT. Results showed that both braces reduced DRUJ mobility in full pronation and supination, with the custom-made brace over-reducing dorsal translation in full pronation. Of note, the braces did not cross the elbow or wrist, thereby allowing full motion, including forearm rotation. This feature of the braces may be particularly useful in patients who have a flat sigmoid notch and bilateral DRUJ hypermobility because their outcomes are unpredictable after reconstructive surgery. In concordance with bracing, a forearm and wrist strengthening program should be instituted.

In those patients in whom nonoperative treatment fails or who do not tolerate brace treatment, the primary indications for DRUJ ligament reconstruction are pain, weakness, clicking, and loss of forearm rotation secondary to distal ulna instability. Contraindications for ligament reconstruction include ulnocarpal impaction and length discrepancies between the radius and the ulna, including untreated malunions, collagen disorders, rheumatoid disease, and frank arthrosis.[24] Chronic DRUJ instability with minimal arthrosis and ulna impaction is best treated with an ulna-shortening osteotomy and ligamentous repair, if the soft tissue sleeve remains loose or unstable after shortening. However, in those patients who have advanced DRUJ arthrosis, salvage procedures such as Sauve-Kapanji procedure, Darrach procedure, or arthroplasty are indicated; these procedures are beyond the scope of this article.

In trying to determine which reconstructive procedure will most likely restore stability and achieve a full, painless range of motion, numerous other factors need to be considered. Ligament reconstruction in the face of a radius and/or ulna malunion is destined to fail unless corrective osteotomies are performed concurrently. In patients who have sigmoid notch incongruity, osteoplasty may be indicated as an adjunct to DRUJ reconstruction, because failure to do so results in persistent instability.[21] Osteoplasty can be performed to recreate the volar or dorsal lip to act as a buttress against dorsopalmar translation.[20,21]

SOFT TISSUE RECONSTRUCTION FOR CHRONIC INSTABILITY

Soft tissue reconstruction of the DRUJ is indicated in the symptomatic patient in whom the TFCC is irreparable and the sigmoid notch competent. Ideally, the reconstruction should link the ulna to the carpus and provide stabilization of the radius on the ulna permitting rotation.[22] However, a reconstruction encompassing all these parameters does not exist. Present treatment of chronic DRUJ instability includes (1) the creation of a radioulnar tether extrinsic to the DRUJ,[30] (2) extensor retinaculum capsulorrhaphy procedure (Herbert sling),[31,32] (3) creation of an indirect connection between the radius and ulna via an ulnocarpal sling or tenodesis procedure,[25,33,34] and (4) reconstruction of the volar and dorsal radioulnar ligaments.[27] TFCC repair has been well described in the literature, and reports by Anderson and colleagues[35] suggest that there is no significant difference between open or arthroscopic repair. However, TFCC repair is usually only possible in an acute or subacute setting, whereas chronic multidirectional instability usually requires more extensive reconstruction.

Extrinsic Radioulnar Tether

In 1978, Fulkerson and Watson[30] described a technique to stabilize the radioulnar relationship by using an extrinsic tether. The technique is similar to the radioulnar ligament reconstruction that has been described.[27] However, the reconstruction is not anatomic, in that the tether is proximal to the TFCC at the level of the ulnar neck. A quarter-inch drill hole is made in the distal radius at the level of the ulnar neck. A long tendon graft is passed through this hole and around the ulnar neck and secured.[30] In the case report, the investigators noted successful stabilization of a case of anterior subluxation without antecedent trauma using this technique. No larger reports are found in the review of the literature, and this technique likely does not offer any advantage over the anatomic radioulnar ligament reconstruction described by Adams and Berger.[27]

Extensor Retinaculum Capsulorrhaphy Procedure

Originally described by Stanley and Herbert to restore DRUJ stability after ulnar head prosthesis insertion for posttraumatic disorders of the DRUJ, the Herbert sling procedure is predicated on the use of an ulnar-based flap of extensor retinaculum to stabilize the DRUJ in both radioulnar and ulnocarpal orientations. The flap is advanced at a 30°- to 40°-angle from distal ulnar to proximal radial and secured into the distal radial periosteum, thereby reducing the DRUJ and carpus to the ulna.[31,32] In brief, a longitudinal incision is centered over the fifth extensor compartment at the level of the wrist. The retinaculum is incised at the junction of the fourth and fifth compartments, with care taken not to enter the fourth compartment. The extensor digiti minimi tendon is retracted radially, and an ulnar-based flap of the retinaculum is raised as it is detached from the ulnar and triquetrum. The often-supinated carpus is then reduced by a combination of carpal pronation and directed pressure on the ulna. The retinacular flap is advanced from distal ulnar to proximal radial and secured to the ulnar border of the distal radial periosteum using 2-0 polydioxanone suture or suture anchors. The extensor digiti minimi tendon is left transposed dorsal to the extensor retinaculum (**Fig. 4**). In their series of 20 Swanson ulnar head prostheses used to treat posttraumatic disorders of the DRUJ, Stanley and Herbert[32] reported good to excellent results in 70% of patients at a mean of 44 months postoperatively. The reported complications were related to implant fracture and synovitis and not to persistent instability, thereby providing support to the Herbert sling procedure as an effective technique to restoring DRUJ stability.

Ulnocarpal Sling (Linscheid-Hui Procedure)

In 1982, Hui and Linscheid[25] conducted a series of cadaveric experiments to determine which structures needed to be reconstructed to reduce dorsopalmar instability. During forearm pronation, the dorsal radioulnar ligaments tightened and the ulna collateral ligament twisted palmarly forming a hammock-like arrangement under the ulna head, displacing it dorsally. The volar structures were lax. When the dorsal restraints were sectioned, the investigators noted dorsal displacement of the ulna head and supination deformity of the radiocarpal joint at the DRUJ, secondary to deforming forces from the ulna collateral ligament. Based on these findings, the investigators devised a volar ulnocarpal ligament reconstructive procedure using a distally based strip of the flexor carpi ulnaris (FCU) tendon.[24,25] In their series of 8 young and active patients, Hui and Linscheid[25] reported excellent results in 5 patients and satisfactory pain relief in 3. All patients were satisfied with the operation, although they all had some loss of pronation.

Surgical technique

With the forearm pronated, a curvilinear incision is made from the midforearm over the subcutaneous border of the ulna, extending distally and dorsally over the ulnocarpal joint (**Fig. 5**). An alternative approach uses a dorsal and volar incision similar to the approach for volar and dorsal radioulnar ligament reconstruction described later. Having identified and protected the dorsal sensory branch of the ulna nerve, a perforation in the volar capsule is made to (**Fig. 6**) permit passage of a 10-cm distally based strip of FCU (**Fig. 7**). Care must be taken to ensure that the underlying ulnar nerve and artery are protected. A 26-gauge wire is tied to the end of the tendon graft to aid in its eventual dorsal passage.

The ulnocarpal joint and distal ulna are exposed by incising the extensor retinaculum in line with the fifth extensor compartment. The retinaculum is elevated off the sixth compartment, with care taken to preserve the ECU subsheath. With the ulnocarpal capsule exposed, a longitudinal arthrotomy is made ensuring that the dorsal radioulnar ligament is not injured. If the TFCC is torn from the ulna styloid, it is repaired at this point.

Using multiplanar fluoroscopy, an oblique bone tunnel is created by passing a 2-mm drill bit from

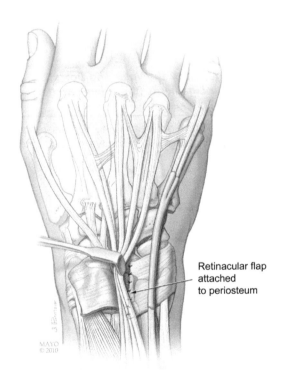

Retinacular flap attached to periosteum

Fig. 4. Herbert sling procedure demonstrating suture fixation of the ulnar-based retinacular flap to the dorsal/ulnar aspect of the distal radius. (*Courtesy of* Mayo Clinic, Rochester, MN; with permission.)

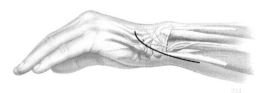

Fig. 5. Curvilinear incision along the subcutaneous border of the distal ulna, extending distally over the base of the fifth metacarpus. (*Courtesy of* Mayo Clinic, Rochester, MN; with permission.)

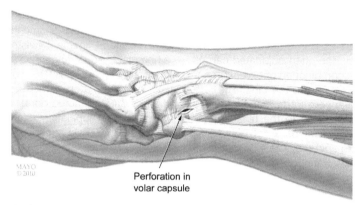

Perforation in
volar capsule

Fig. 6. A perforation in the pisotriquetral ligament is made on the volar capsule to aid in the passage of the FCU tendon. (*Courtesy of* Mayo Clinic, Rochester, MN; with permission.)

the dorsal ulna neck to the fovea of the distal ulna (see **Fig. 7**). The drill is removed and the tunnel serially dilated up to 4 to 5 mm with hand awls. The FCU tendon graft is then passed from a volar to dorsal direction, with care taken to ensure that the ulnar neurovascular bundle is not impinged. As the tendon exits dorsally, it is pulled taut either through the TFCC or distal to the TFCC and then through the bone tunnel within the distal ulna. This construct creates a volar reduction force on the ulna head, thereby reducing any dorsal instability (**Fig. 8**). The capsular incisions are closed with 3-0 nonabsorbable sutures. To neutralize the deforming forces on the soft tissue construct, the forearm is supinated and provisional DRUJ reduction is held with 2 parallel 0.0625 in Kirschner (K) wires. The tendon graft is pulled tight and secured to the periosteum with nonabsorbable 2-0 sutures. The graft is then folded over itself and sewn to its proximal limb or to the pisotriquetral ligament (**Fig. 9**). The

retinaculum is closed with 3-0 nonabsorbable sutures and the tourniquet is deflated. Once hemostasis is obtained, the wounds are closed and the patient's wrist is placed into a long arm splint. On the first postoperative day, digital range of motion and edema control are initiated. At 2 weeks after surgery, the sutures are removed and the patient's arm is placed in a long arm cast or Munster cast for an additional 4 weeks, at which point the K wires are removed and the patient is placed in a custom-molded ulna gutter splint. Gentle motion is initiated and gradually increased over a period of 3 to 4 months under the guidance of a hand therapist.

Reconstruction of the Volar and Dorsal Radioulnar Ligaments (the Adams-Berger Procedure)

Despite the development of the various reconstructive techniques, studies have demonstrated

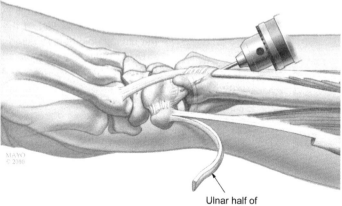

Ulnar half of
Flexor Carpi Ulnaris tendon

Fig. 7. An oblique bone tunnel is made within the distal ulna from the dorsal ulna to the fovea. (*Courtesy of* Mayo Clinic, Rochester, MN; with permission.)

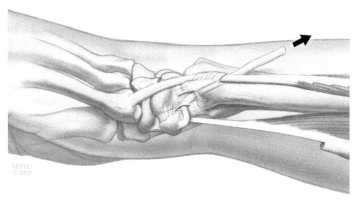

Fig. 8. The FCU tendon graft is delivered through the pisotriquetral arthrotomy, the TFCC, and oblique bone tunnel to create a volar reduction force on the distal ulna. (*Courtesy of* Mayo Clinic, Rochester, MN; with permission.)

significant biomechanical deficiencies in the ability to stabilize the DRUJ. Petersen and Adams[36] demonstrated that both the radioulnar sling and tenodesis procedures failed to restore natural joint stability. Despite the sling procedure being more stable than tenodesis, the investigators noted that the radioulnar tether at the level of the ulnar neck did not permit movement of the forearm along its normal axis of rotation and that the ulnocarpal sling procedures became lax with time. With these findings in mind, rather than reconstructing the ulnocarpal ligaments, Adams and Berger[27] described a technique that reconstructs the anatomic origin and insertion of the palmar and dorsal radioulnar ligaments.[37,38]

Surgical technique

A longitudinal incision is made between the fifth and sixth extensor compartments. The fifth compartment is opened and the extensor digiti minimi retracted radially. The ECU sheath is left untouched within the ulna groove. An L-shaped DRUJ capsulotomy is made with one limb along the dorsal rim of the sigmoid notch and the other just proximal to the dorsal radioulnar ligament.

Subperiosteal dissection is performed from the dorsal margin of the sigmoid notch under the fourth extensor compartment. This dissection enables passage of a guidewire that is to be placed through the distal radius, 5 mm proximal to the lunate facet and 5 mm radial to the articular surface of the sigmoid notch. A 3.5-mm cannulated drill bit is then passed over the guidewire to create the radial bone tunnel. Using a similar cannulated system, an ulna bone tunnel is created between the fovea and the ulna neck (**Fig. 10**).

Then a longitudinal incision of 4 cm is made on the volar aspect of the wrist between the ulna neurovascular bundle and the flexor tendons to expose the radial tunnel. One end of a free tendon graft (eg, palmaris longus, plantaris, toe extensor, FCU, or a strip of flexor carpi radialis) is delivered dorsally through this bony tunnel and the other end is passed over the ulna head, proximal to the TFCC, through the volar DRUJ capsule. In this way, both ends of the tendon graft are delivered dorsally and then passed through the ulna tunnel. The limbs are then passed in opposite directions around the ulna neck, one limb lying deep to the ECU (**Fig. 11**). Before tensioning the

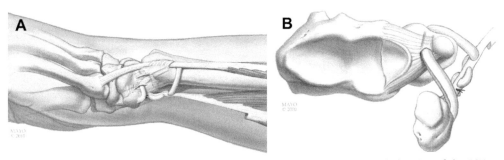

Fig. 9. (*A, B*) Two-view drawing demonstrating closure of the DRUJ arthrotomy and plication of the FCU tendon graft onto its proximal limb. (*Courtesy of* Mayo Clinic, Rochester, MN; with permission.)

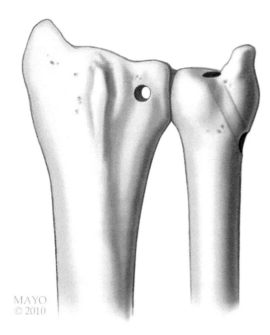

Fig. 10. Location of radial and ulnar bone tunnels for volar and dorsal radioulnar ligament reconstruction of the fovea. (*Courtesy of* Mayo Clinic, Rochester, MN; with permission.)

reconstruction, the forearm is placed in neutral rotation and the DRUJ manually compressed. The limbs are pulled tight, tied together, and secured with 3-0 nonabsorbable sutures (see **Fig. 11**). The capsule of the dorsal DRUJ and extensor retinaculum (extensor digiti minimi left free) are closed in layers with 3-0 sutures. The patient's arm is placed in a Munster cast for 6 weeks, followed by a removable Munster splint with a gradual and progressive gentle active range of motion exercise program for an additional 4

weeks. Under the supervision of a hand therapist, the patient is allowed to perform active wrist motion, gentle hand and forearm strengthening, and active forearm rotation. Passive exercises are restricted, and the patient usually regains pronation and supination over 4 to 6 months. Heavy lifting and impact loading are permitted after 6 months.

Outcomes

Adams and Berger[27] reported their experience in 14 patients over a 4-year period. Subjectively, 9 patients were pain free, 3 improved, and 2 showed no change. DRUJ stability was noted in 12 patients, all of whom returned to their previous occupation or sports without restrictions. There were 2 patients who developed some recurrence of DRUJ instability: one had a deficient palmar rim of the sigmoid notch and the other had evidence of carpal supination deformity.

With palmaris longus as the tendon graft of choice, Seo and colleagues[39] reported their experience using the Adams-Berger technique. A total of 16 patients with subluxation or DRUJ instability after trauma were followed up for a mean period of 18.9 months. The investigators found that 11 patients had volar instability and 5 had dorsal instability. Ten patients underwent concomitant corrective osteotomy for malunion of their radial fracture in conjunction to the tenodesis procedure. Results demonstrated normal dorsopalmar stability in 12 patients, mild laxity in 3, and residual subluxation in 1. Using the modified Mayo wrist score, excellent results were reported in 10 patients, good results in 5, and poor outcome in 1. Average grip strength improved from 31 to 36 kg. An additional secondary osteotomy was performed in 1 patient with residual subluxation.[39]

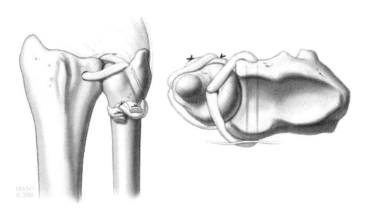

Fig. 11. Passage of the free tendon graft through the radial and ulnar bone tunnels and around the ulna neck, and securing of the graft with permanent suture. (*Courtesy of* Mayo Clinic, Rochester, MN; with permission.)

Similar results were reported by Teoh and Yam.[40] At an average of 9 years postreconstruction, the average Mayo wrist score was 87, with joint stability being maintained in 7 of 9 patients. Possible causes for residual joint laxity in the remaining 2 patients were insufficient tensioning of the graft and rupture or loosening of the graft during initial mobilization. Compared with their preoperative examination, total forearm rotation decreased from 169° to 155°. Average grip strength improved and was maintained over the long term. Follow-up radiographs demonstrated no DRUJ or ulnocarpal joint degeneration.[40]

SUMMARY

Chronic instability of the DRUJ can be a common cause of ulna-sided wrist pain. In cases of chronic instability, repair of the TFCC may not be possible, necessitating formal ligament reconstruction provided there is no evidence of concomitant arthrosis of the sigmoid notch. If the arthrosis is present, ligament reconstruction should be abandoned in favor of DRUJ arthroplasty or some other salvage technique.

REFERENCES

1. Johnston K, Durand D, Hildebrand KA. Chronic volar distal radioulnar joint instability: joint capsular plication to restore function. Can J Surg 2009; 52(2):112–8.
2. Ray RD, Johnson RJ, Jameson RM. Rotation of the forearm; an experimental study of pronation and supination. J Bone Joint Surg Am 1951;33(4):993–6.
3. Stuart PR, Berger RA, Linscheid RL, et al. The dorsopalmar stability of the distal radioulnar joint. J Hand Surg Am 2000;25(4):689–99.
4. Tolat AR, Stanley JK, Trail IA. A cadaveric study of the anatomy and stability of the distal radioulnar joint in the coronal and transverse planes. J Hand Surg Br 1996;21(5):587–94.
5. af Ekenstam F, Hagert CG. Anatomical studies on the geometry and stability of the distal radio ulnar joint. Scand J Plast Reconstr Surg 1985; 19(1):17–25.
6. Kihara H, Short WH, Werner FW, et al. The stabilizing mechanism of the distal radioulnar joint during pronation and supination. J Hand Surg Am 1995; 20(6):930–6.
7. Schuind F, An KN, Berglund L, et al. The distal radioulnar ligaments: a biomechanical study. J Hand Surg Am 1991;16(6):1106–14.
8. Ward LD, Ambrose CG, Masson MV, et al. The role of the distal radioulnar ligaments, interosseous membrane, and joint capsule in distal radioulnar joint stability. J Hand Surg Am 2000;25(2):341–51.
9. Gofton WT, Gordon KD, Dunning CE, et al. Soft-tissue stabilizers of the distal radioulnar joint: an in vitro kinematic study. J Hand Surg Am 2004;29(3):423–31.
10. Garcia-Elias M. Soft-tissue anatomy and relationships about the distal ulna. Hand Clin 1998;14(2):165–76.
11. Lindau T. Treatment of injuries to the ulnar side of the wrist occurring with distal radial fractures. Hand Clin 2005;21(3):417–25.
12. Fontes D, Lenoble E, de Somer B, et al. [Lesions of the ligaments associated with distal fractures of the radius. 58 intraoperative arthrographies]. Ann Chir Main Memb Super 1992;11(2):119–25 [in French].
13. Mohanti RC, Kar N. Study of triangular fibrocartilage of the wrist joint in Colles' fracture. Injury 1980;11(4):321–4.
14. Geissler WB, Freeland AE, Savoie FH, et al. Intracarpal soft-tissue lesions associated with an intra-articular fracture of the distal end of the radius. J Bone Joint Surg Am 1996;78(3):357–65.
15. Lindau T, Adlercreutz C, Aspenberg P. Peripheral tears of the triangular fibrocartilage complex cause distal radioulnar joint instability after distal radial fractures. J Hand Surg Am 2000;25(3):464–8.
16. Kim JK, Koh YD, Do NH. Should an ulnar styloid fracture be fixed following volar plate fixation of a distal radial fracture? J Bone Joint Surg Am 2010;92(1):1–6.
17. Frykman G. Fracture of the distal radius including sequelae–shoulder-hand-finger syndrome, disturbance in the distal radio-ulnar joint and impairment of nerve function. A clinical and experimental study. Acta Orthop Scand 1967;(Suppl 108):3+.
18. Knirk JL, Jupiter JB. Intra-articular fractures of the distal end of the radius in young adults. J Bone Joint Surg Am 1986;68(5):647–59.
19. Oskarsson GV, Aaser P, Hjall A. Do we underestimate the predictive value of the ulnar styloid affection in Colles fractures? Arch Orthop Trauma Surg 1997;116(6–7):341–4.
20. Adams BD. Effects of radial deformity on distal radioulnar joint mechanics. J Hand Surg Am 1993; 18:492–8.
21. Kihara H, Palmer AK, Werner FW, et al. The effect of dorsally angulated distal radius fractures on distal radioulnar joint congruency and forearm rotation. J Hand Surg Am 1996;21:40–7.
22. Rettig ME, Raskin KB. Galeazzi fracture-dislocation: a new treatment-oriented classification. J Hand Surg Am 2001;26(2):228–35.
23. Tay SC, Tomita K, Berger RA. The "ulnar fovea sign" for defining ulnar wrist pain: an analysis of sensitivity and specificity. J Hand Surg Am 2007;32(4):438–44.
24. Glowacki KA, Shin LA. Stabilization of the unstable distal ulna: the Linscheid-Hui procedure. Tech Hand Up Extrem Surg 1999;3(4):229–36.
25. Hui FC, Linscheid RL. Ulnotriquetral augmentation tenodesis: a reconstructive procedure for dorsal

subluxation of the distal radioulnar joint. J Hand Surg Am 1982;7(3):230–6.

26. Lester B, Halbrecht J, Levy IM, et al. Press test" for office diagnosis of triangular fibrocartilage complex tears of the wrist. Ann Plast Surg 1995;35(1):41–5.

27. Adams BD, Berger RA. An anatomic reconstruction of the distal radioulnar ligaments for posttraumatic distal radioulnar joint instability. J Hand Surg Am 2002;27(2):243–51.

28. Tay SC, Berger RA, Tomita K, et al. In vivo three-dimensional displacement of the distal radioulnar joint during resisted forearm rotation. J Hand Surg Am 2007;32(4):450–8.

29. Millard GM, Budoff JE, Paravic V, et al. Functional bracing for distal radioulnar joint instability. J Hand Surg Am 2002;27(6):972–7.

30. Fulkerson JP, Watson HK. Congenital anterior subluxation of the distal ulna. A case report. Clin Orthop Relat Res 1978;(131):179–82.

31. Dy CJ, Ouellette EA, Makowski AL. Extensor retinaculum capsulorrhaphy for ulnocarpal and distal radioulnar instability: the Herbert sling. Tech Hand Up Extrem Surg 2009;13(1):19–22.

32. Stanley D, Herbert TJ. The Swanson ulnar head prosthesis for post-traumatic disorders of the distal radio-ulnar joint. J Hand Surg Br 1992;17(6):682–8.

33. Breen TF, Jupiter JB. Extensor carpi ulnaris and flexor carpi ulnaris tenodesis of the unstable distal ulna. J Hand Surg Am 1989;14(4):612–7.

34. Tsai TM, Stilwell JH. Repair of chronic subluxation of the distal radioulnar joint (ulnar dorsal) using flexor carpi ulnaris tendon. J Hand Surg Br 1984; 9(3):289–94.

35. Anderson ML, Larson AN, Moran SL, et al. Clinical comparison of arthroscopic versus open repair of triangular fibrocartilage complex tears. J Hand Surg Am 2008;33(5):675–82.

36. Petersen MS, Adams BD. Biomechanical evaluation of distal radioulnar reconstructions. J Hand Surg Am 1993;18(2):328–34.

37. Adams BD, Lawler E. Chronic instability of the distal radioulnar joint. J Am Acad Orthop Surg 2007;15(9): 571–5.

38. Lawler E, Adams BD. Reconstruction for DRUJ instability. Hand (N Y) 2007;2(3):123–6.

39. Seo KN, Park MJ, Kang HJ. Anatomic reconstruction of the distal radioulnar ligament for posttraumatic distal radioulnar joint instability. Clin Orthop Surg 2009;1(3):138–45.

40. Teoh LC, Yam AK. Anatomic reconstruction of the distal radioulnar ligaments: long-term results. J Hand Surg Br 2005;30(2):185–93.

Salvage of Failed Distal Radioulnar Joint Reconstruction

Adam C. Watts, FRCS (Tr and Ortho)*,
Michael J. Hayton, FRCS (Tr and Ortho), FFSEM(UK),
John K. Stanley, FRCS, FRCSEd

KEYWORDS
• DRUJ • Reconstruction • Failed • Salvage

Painful arthrosis of the distal radioulnar joint (DRUJ) is multifactorial and may arise because of trauma, primary osteoarthrosis, inflammatory arthritis, crystal deposition disease, or infection. There are several options for treatment, including a Darrach resection arthroplasty, matched hemiresection with or without interposition, and Sauve-Kapanji procedure. The outcome of these procedures is unpredictable, and, if they fail, they may present a significant surgical challenge. When planning salvage options, it is important to first consider the normal anatomy and biomechanics of the joint and then the primary procedures that are performed and their indications as well as to understand the modes of failure. Thus, it may be possible to determine why a procedure has failed, and strategies for salvage reconstruction can be developed.

ANATOMY OF DRUJ

The DRUJ cannot be considered in isolation but should be considered an articulation with the forearm joint. The forearm has 2 radioulnar articulations separated by a fixed strut, the ulna, from which the radius is suspended by the central condensation of the interosseous membrane and around which the radius rotates.[1] In this sense, the forearm can be considered, like the knee joint, as a bicondylar articulation separated by a nonarticulating segment, which contains the primary ligamentous restraint. The ability to pronate and supinate, afforded by this articulation, has allowed our ancestors to swing through the trees in fight or flight, and humans to exploit the potential of the hand with an opposable thumb to manipulate tools.

The DRUJ has 2 components: the osseous radioulnar articulation and the ligamentous attachments of the distal ulna. The articular portion of the ulna head within the DRUJ is known as the seat, and this articulates with the sigmoid notch of the radius. There is a mismatch in the radius of curvature of these opposing surfaces. The articular cartilage covers 90° to 135° of the circumference of the ulna head, with an average radius of curvature of 10 mm. The sigmoid notch has an average radius of curvature of 15 mm and occupies a sector of 47° to 80°.[2] The shape and orientation of the sigmoid notch relative to the long axis of the forearm is variable and may be related to the relative ulna length.[3] In most of the population, who are ulna minus, the notch tends to be inclined in a proximal radial to distal ulna direction on a posteroanterior (PA) radiograph; in those who are ulna plus, the opposite holds, with a distal radial orientation; and in those with a neutral ulna, the notch is orientated close to the long axis of the forearm.[4] In addition, Forstner[5] has reported that in the ulnar-minus DRUJ, the notch tends to be conical; in ulna plus, hemispherical; and in ulna neutral, cylindrical.

When considering the movement of the DRUJ, it is unavoidable to consider the movement of the ulna seat within the sigmoid notch; of course, in truth, the radius rotates around the ulna, which is

Upper Limb Unit, Wrightington Hospital, Hall Lane, Appley Bridge, Wigan, WN6 9EP, UK
* Corresponding author.
E-mail address: adamcwatts@hotmail.com

Hand Clin 26 (2010) 529–541
doi:10.1016/j.hcl.2010.05.004
0749-0712/10/$ – see front matter © 2010 Elsevier Inc. All rights reserved.

fixed proximally to the humerus. The sigmoid notch not only rotates around the ulna seat during pronation and supination but also translates relative to the long axis of the ulna in the ventral-dorsal and the proximal-distal vectors. At the extremes of forearm rotation, the contact area of the articular surfaces is only 2 to 3 mm.[2]

The stabilizers of the DRUJ can be considered in 2 groups: (1) the static stabilizers (elements of the triangular fibrocartilaginous complex [TFCC], the joint capsule, and the distal portion of the interosseous membrane) and (2) the dynamic stabilizers (extensor carpi ulnaris [ECU], pronator quadratus, and supinator). The TFCC consists of the fibrocartilaginous articular disk bound by the radius, the dorsal and volar radioulnar ligaments, and the sheath of the ECU.[6] The radioulnar ligaments have 2 elements: a superficial bundle from which the disk is suspended and deep elements, the primary stabilizers of the DRUJ, that converge proximally and ulnarward to attach to the fovea on the head of the ulna.

The DRUJ can be approached from the dorsal, volar, or subcutaneous border of the ulna. The dorsal approach allows the surgeon to preserve a strong capsular layer for reconstruction and is the authors' preferred approach. A curvilinear dorsal incision is made over the fifth extensor compartment, which is approached from the radial side of the tendon. The floor of the compartment is incised to enter the DRUJ, ensuring that a cuff of tissue is left attached to the radius for later repair. An ulnar-based L- or U-shaped flap can be elevated with the careful preservation of the dorsal radioulnar ligament of the TFCC. This flap is robust and can be repaired satisfactorily at the end of the procedure. A retrospective review of 55 patients who underwent surgery through this approach revealed only 1 complication, that of neuroma formation secondary to injury to the dorsal sensory branch of the ulnar nerve.[7]

BIOMECHANICS OF DRUJ

Forearm rotation of 150° occurs at the DRUJ, with the radius describing an arc of rotation around the center of the ulna head. This movement is complex and is coupled with proximal translation in pronation and with dorsal and ulna translation. At the same time, the ulna head moves in space by up to 9° from a valgus position in pronation to a more varus position in supination.[8]

In full pronation, the radius translates, so that the dorsal lip of the sigmoid notch articulates with the seat of the ulna and is limited by tension within the deep element of the volar radioulnar ligament. In full supination, the radius translates,

so that the volar lip of the sigmoid notch contacts the seat of the ulna and the tension is transferred to the dorsal radioulnar ligament.

However, according to Stuart and colleagues,[9] the fact that these structures reach their maximum length in the positions described earlier does not mean that they are acting as restraints. From their serial sectioning study in fresh-frozen cadavers, these investigators concluded that the palmar radioulnar ligament is the primary restraint against volar translation of the radius relative to the ulna in all positions of the wrist. Dorsal translation restraint seems to be shared by the palmar and dorsal radioulnar ligaments and the interosseous membrane.[9] Further, the investigators argue that 20% of the restraint is caused by radioulnar contact.

This movement can thus be summarized as follows: as the wrist moves from full supination to pronation, the radius glides around the ulna head in an arc from dorsal distal to palmar proximal, while the ulna itself moves from a varus to valgus position.

Palmer and Werner[10] have also shown that approximately 80% of the load through the intact wrist is borne by the radius and 20% by the ulna through the TFCC. Radial deviation of the wrist, as is seen in power grip, increases the proportion of the load that is transferred to the radius. Serial sectioning studies performed by the same investigators confirmed that the TFCC, interosseous membrane, and pronator quadratus are important stabilizers of the DRUJ.[10]

PRIMARY PROCEDURES FOR DRUJ ARTHROSIS

Several procedures have been described to tackle pain or restriction of movement arising from arthrosis of the DRUJ. The most commonly performed procedure is the Darrach resection arthroplasty. Excision of the ulna head is performed to the level of the proximal extent of the sigmoid notch. Variable outcomes have been reported in the literature after Darrach procedure, with satisfactory outcomes ranging from 50% to 91% for posttrauma pathology.[11–13] Among 95 cases of rheumatoid wrists, the outcomes were reported to be good or excellent in only 67%, using American Rheumatology Association Therapeutic Criteria.[14]

Concerns have been expressed in the literature about problems with forearm instability and radioulnar impingement.[15] George reported that after Darrach resection some patients had pain with forearm rotation on power grip, such as when wringing out clothes, and 2 patients had clicking during forearm rotation. Field and colleagues[11] reported radioulnar convergence in 9 of 36 patients who underwent Darrach resection and pain in 31 patients (22 on pronosupination and 20 on power grip). Sixteen patients in their series had clicking and stiffness. On examination, 50% had pain on resisted supination, 17 of 36 had pain on radioulnar compression, and 18 of 36 had pain on piano key test. Twenty-nine patients had significantly reduced grip strength. Radiological examination revealed ulna translation of the carpus in at least 22 of 36 cases, and 17 of 36 cases had signs of scalloping of the radius. Patient satisfaction was statistically related to grip strength, increased ulna resection, and radiographic signs of osteoarthritis.[11]

In an attempt to address the radioulnar instability, many variations to the Darrach procedure have been described, including limited or domed resection, tendon stabilization, and interposition, but overall results are similar to the original procedure.[16–18] Other alternative procedures such as the Sauve-Kapanji procedure and the matched distal ulna hemiresection with or without interposition have equal and unpredictable outcomes that are similar to the Darrach procedure.[7,15,19]

MODES OF FAILURE OF PRIMARY DRUJ PROCEDURES

Investigators have subsequently sought explanation for why some patients have no problem after ulnar head resection, whereas others develop painful forearm instability. Bieber and colleagues[20] performed a review of 20 patients with pain and limitation of activities at a minimum of 29 months (29–135 months, average 61 months) after ulnar head resection. In a search for a possible cause, they undertook a review of postoperative radiographs. The investigators were unable to detect any radiographic differences from those who had had a successful Darrach procedure. In their experience, reoperation to restore forearm stability was rarely successful.[20] McKee and Richards[21] drew a different conclusion. They reviewed 23 of 30 patients after they had Darrach procedure, with a follow-up of 36 to 121 months (average 75.5 months). Among the 23 patients, 19 were satisfied with their outcome, but 7 had pain with mild or heavy activity. Difficult tasks included lifting heavy objects (13 of 23 patients), opening jars (8 of 23), and turning doorknobs (7 of 23). When examined, 4 patients had pain on resisted forearm rotation and 4 patients on distal radioulnar compression; all the 8 patients had radiographic signs of distal radioulnar impingement. The investigators examined

the anteroposterior (AP) and lateral radiographs of the forearm taken at rest and power grip. From these radiographs, they were able to quantify dynamic radioulnar convergence and radioulnar impingement. Dynamic radioulnar convergence was seen in 14 patients (56%). Of these 14 patients, 5 had radioulnar impingement with visible scalloping and sclerosis, but only 2 of these patients were symptomatic. However, they did report that dynamic radioulnar convergence correlated with increased amount of resection of distal ulna and concluded that the incidence of radioulnar impingement was 8% and associated with a larger ulna resection. The investigators postulated that dynamic radioulnar convergence is caused by the pull of the muscles that cross the wrist, with some crossing from the radius in the forearm to the ulnar side of the hand (ECU) and others going from the ulna to the radial side of the hand (flexor digitorum profundus to index and middle finger, flexor pollicis longus) in the absence of the distal forearm condyle, the ulna head.

Bell and colleagues[22] coined the term ulnar impingement syndrome. In a group of 11 patients with a shortened ulna either after resection or after growth arrest, they described a collection of symptoms of a painful wrist with weak grip and clicking on pronation or supination. Pain was exacerbated in all cases by pushing the radius and ulna together. Pronosupination reproduced a painful click, and the pain intensified with resisted supination. The distal stump was unstable in the AP plane, and grip strength was markedly reduced. The investigators described 3 appearances on a PA radiograph of the wrist: a shortened ulna, radioulnar convergence, and scalloping of the radius at the level of the tip of the ulna resection. The investigators stated that after distal ulna resection, "radio-ulnar convergence is inevitable," and they attributed this to the actions of extensor pollicis brevis, abductor pollicis longus, and pronator quadratus and to the effect of the interosseous membrane. To this the authors add the effect of gravity when the arm is held in neutral rotation with the shoulder adducted and elbow flexed to 90°, especially with loading, such as when carrying a cup or jug. The investigators concluded that in cases of traumatic dysfunction of the DRUJ, reconstruction is preferable to ulna head excision.

These clinical studies are supported by data from cadaveric experiments that have also demonstrated the destabilizing effect of resection of the ulna head. Sauerbier and colleagues[23] performed a dynamic test on 7 cadaveric limbs, with loading of individual muscle groups using a simulator. The investigators concluded that ulna head resection creates extensive forearm instability with displacement of the radius toward the ulna. From the simulation, they were able to demonstrate that distal ulna prosthetic replacement restores some stability, but dorsopalmar displacement may occur either after ulna head resection or after replacement. The same investigators compared matched hemiresection with Darrach resection arthroplasty using the same simulator.[24] In this study, the matched hemiresection arthroplasty demonstrated less radioulnar convergence than Darrach arthroplasty, presumably because more of the soft tissue restraints are preserved.

One reason for the different conclusions of the previous studies is that both studies were focusing on the element that can be seen on radiographs, namely the extent of ulna resection, and were ignoring the soft tissue pathology. It is likely that there is significant variability in the pathologic condition of the stabilizers around the DRUJ. The serial sectioning studies reported earlier demonstrate that loss of 1 restraint alone may be insufficient to result in instability, but there is an additive effect. In some joints, although the articular surface may be destroyed, the restraining soft tissues may be relatively preserved; in others, the static and dynamic stabilizers may have been significantly disrupted by trauma, synovitis, or previous surgical intervention. Therefore, removing an additional stabilizer is destined to result in further instability. For example, a large proportion of the pathologic conditions of the DRUJ is seen in conjunction with a distal radius fracture; it is likely in many cases that coincident disruption of the TFCC or distal interosseous membrane has occurred at the time of injury, a feature that is often not well documented in assessment of distal radius fractures. Surgical intervention to the radius may add further to the insult to the dynamic stabilizers of the DRUJ, with the disruption of the pronator quadratus and brachioradialis (that may help suspend the radius when the forearm is loaded in neutral rotation, with the shoulder adducted and the elbow flexed to 90°), as well as to the static elements such as the volar radiolunate ligament and volar joint capsule.

INVESTIGATIONS FOR FAILED DRUJ SURGERY

When faced with a patient with persistent or exacerbated symptoms after DRUJ surgery, it is important to document the primary complaint (pain, clicking, limited forearm rotation, reduced grip) and what precipitates or exacerbates these symptoms. A careful exploration of the initial indication for surgery and previous surgical interventions may give some clue as to the cause of the problem. The forearm should be carefully assessed clinically and radiographically. Swelling and deformity in all positions of forearm rotation and, likewise, the stability of the distal ulna in full pronation, neutral rotation, and full supination should be documented. If the DRUJ is found to be unstable, the wrist should be placed in radial deviation to determine whether tightening the ulnar-sided structures restores stability (C. Heras-Palou, MD, personal communication, 2005). Compression applied to the distal radius and ulna with forearm rotation may elicit pain. Standard plain AP and lateral radiographs of the wrist and forearm should be obtained. These radiographs may show evidence of scalloping of the distal radius and sclerosis. In addition, a Scheker view is useful to evaluate radio-ulnar impingement.[25] The wrist is stressed by asking the patient to hold a 2.2-kg lead cylinder, with the shoulder adducted and the elbow flexed to 90° and the forearm in neutral rotation. The radiograph is then taken with the beam in the coronal plane with respect to the anatomic position (**Fig. 1**). In some cases, computed tomography of the distal radius may reveal disruption of the anatomy of the sigmoid notch, such that it presents a flat surface or, in some cases, a convex surface with an absent dorsal lip that may contribute to instability, especially after distal ulna reconstruction procedures.

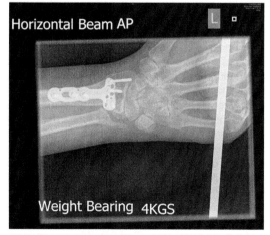

Fig. 1. Scheker view of the DRUJ demonstrating radioulnar impingement on loading. (*From* Lees VC, Scheker LR. The radiological demonstration of dynamic ulnar impingement. J Hand Surg Br 1997;22:448–50; with permission.)

SALVAGE OPTIONS

The first line of surgical treatment that can be considered to salvage the failed DRUJ surgery can involve reconstruction of soft tissue stabilizers, increased osseous constraint, or prosthetic replacement. For those with persistent symptoms after these interventions, the true salvage procedures include wide resection or creation of a one-bone forearm. These procedures are discussed in the following sections.

Tendon Stabilization and Interposition

Breen and Jupiter[26] described a technique using a combined ECU/flexor carpi ulnaris (FCU) tenodesis to provide stabilization of an unstable distal ulna in 8 patients. Among them, 3 patients had had previous distal ulna resection and 5 with intact but degenerate DRUJ had had distal ulna excision and ECU/FCU tenodesis. The technique involves a dorsal and volar approach to the ECU and FCU, respectively. Half of ECU is harvested as a proximally based graft, and half of FCU is harvested as a distally based graft. A drill hole is made in the distal ulna stump from distal volar to proximal dorsal direction. A further drill hole is passed from the cut surface of the ulna to meet the transverse drill hole in the medullary cavity. The grafts are passed through the drill hole, with the FCU graft entering the hole on the cut surface of the ulna and exiting dorsally and the ECU graft passing from the dorsal to the volar hole in the ulna. With the forearm in supination, the grafts are pulled tight and sutured to each other with a nonabsorbable suture. The ECU tendon is stabilized with a pulley that is constructed with part of the extensor retinaculum. The limb is immobilized in supination for 6 weeks. At a minimum follow-up of 18 months (18–63 months, average 28 months), all patients had a stable distal ulna with increased forearm rotation. Seven of the 8 patients had returned to their previous level of work and 1 patient developed complex regional pain syndrome.

Tsai and Stilwell[27] performed a similar technique using a distally based FCU graft passed through the cut end of the ulna, out through a dorsal drill hole, through the interosseous membrane, and around the ECU before being sutured to itself. Five patients reviewed at a minimum of 6 months had satisfactory outcomes, but 1 patient developed a click on forearm rotation and required ulnar nerve decompression at the wrist.[27]

A further soft tissue stabilization described by Johnson,[28] uses the pronator quadratus to act as a dynamic tether for the unstable DRUJ. The pronator quadratus origin is elevated from the distal ulna with subperiosteal dissection. The forearm is pronated, and the pronator quadratus is advanced dorsally between the radius and ulna and is then sutured to the ECU sheath. The forearm was held in neutral rotation with 2 Kirschner (K) wires, crosspinning the radius and ulna for 4 weeks. It was stated that this procedure successfully corrected dorsal instability with a minimum follow-up of 2 years. A further series reported on the long-term outcome (range 5–9 years, average 8 years) of pronator quadratus interposition, as part of a primary Darrach procedure (8 patients) or for the treatment of a failed Darrach procedure (7 patients). Five patients from the original series of 20 patients were lost to follow-up. The investigators reported mixed results, with loss of forearm rotation and reduction but not the complete elimination of pain in the group in which Darrach procedure failed. Three patients, 1 from the primary group and 2 from the secondary group, required salvage with the one-bone forearm procedure.[29] In vitro loading studies that compared Breen and Jupiter's method of stabilization with pronator quadratus interposition demonstrate that radioulnar convergence produced by distal ulna resection is not prevented by either procedure in cadaveric specimens. Under some conditions, the pronator quadratus interposition actually exacerbated the problem.[30]

An alternative to pronator quadratus interposition is the dynamic brachioradialis sling described by Shah and Klimisch.[31] The brachioradialis tendon is transected at the muscle-tendon junction and mobilized to its insertion at the radial styloid. The graft is passed deep to the pronator quadratus so that it maintains contact with the distal radius, and on the ulnar border of the radius it is delivered dorsally around the ulnar stump beneath the ECU. The graft is then woven through FCU with enough tension to elevate the radius while the forearm is held in pronation.

Kleinman and Greenberg[32] have reported on a procedure that combines interposition, tendon stabilization, and K-wire fixation. Six patients were reviewed for a minimum of 11 months (11–39 months, average 20 months). The procedure incorporates a pronator quadratus interposition, with distally based ECU tenodesis and K-wire fixation of the distal radius and ulna and with the forearm in neutral rotation and the bones held apart by lamina spreaders. Divergence of the K wires prevents migration of the radius and ulna. The arm is splinted for 6 weeks in a long arm cast. The investigators reported improvement in pain scores, grip strength, and range of pronation and supination. Of the 5 patients with pain at rest before surgery, 1 had no pain postoperatively, 2 had pain only on heavy activity, and 2 had pain on light activities. Three patients returned to their previous level of activity.

If there is deficiency of the joint capsule contributing to distal ulna instability either secondary to synovitis or previous surgery, then soft tissue reconstruction can be a challenge. Berger and Cooney[33] have described a reconstruction technique using Achilles tendon allograft. Through dorsal and palmar approaches, the strip of fascia is secured to the dorsal and palmar rims of the sigmoid notch with as much tension as possible using bone anchors passing deep to the FCU and ECU tendons.[33]

Another technique that uses allograft to maintain the gap between the distal ulna stump and the radius has been described. Sotereanos and colleagues[34] reported on 4 patients with incapacitating pain over the distal stump of the ulna, which increased with active grip, passive compression of the distal radius against the ulna, or on pronation and supination, whereby bulk allograft was interposed between the ulna stump and the radius (**Fig. 2**). Patients were followed up for a minimum of 14 months (14–34 months, average 26 months). Subperiosteal dissection was performed around the neck of the ulna stump up to 6 cm proximal to the cut surface through the previously incised 5/6 interspace. The ulna border of the radius was exposed over the same region, and 2 to 3 suture anchors were placed in the bone. These were used to secure a bulk allograft of human Achilles tendon, with the sutures passing through the ulna stump. The arm was put through an arc of pronation or supination with compression to ensure smooth movement without impingement before layered closure. The arm was splinted for 6 weeks in neutral rotation before rehabilitation. Three of 4 patients

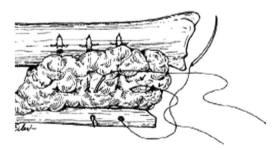

Fig. 2. Allograft interposition procedure described by Sotereanos. (*From* Sotereanos DG, Gobel F, Vardakas DG, et al. An allograft salvage technique for failure of the Darrach procedure: a report of four cases. J Hand Surg Br 2002;27:317; with permission.)

had excellent results, with 1 failure caused by inadequate bulk of graft placed between the bones.[34]

Autograft Osseous Reconstruction

Watson and Brown,[35] encouraged by the early reports of favorable outcomes after matched hemiresection, developed a technique to essentially convert a failed Darrach procedure to a matched hemiresection by advancing part of the distal ulna with a step-cut and shaping the advanced part to match the distal radius. The TFCC and ulnar sling mechanism was attached to the advanced distal ulna. Three case reports were presented with a follow-up of 7, 9, and 24 months, respectively, with outcomes described by the investigators as good.[35] A similar technique described by Hove and Helland[36] used an intercalary tricortical iliac crest autograft. The distal end of the ulna was osteotomized and advanced distally, the osteotomy site was filled with the tricortical graft, and a plate was applied to the construct. Pronator quadratus was brought dorsally between the 2 forearm bones and anchored to the medial periosteum of the ulna and ECU. A longitudinal distally based ECU tenodesis was also performed. The investigators described a satisfactory outcome in 1 patient who presented with loss of forearm rotation and pain.[36]

Similarly, the failed Sauve-Kapanji procedure can be converted to a matched hemiresection using a technique described by Ross and colleagues.[37] The investigators report that in a series of 71 Sauve-Kapanji procedures, 6 patients developed painful stump instability. The investigators surmised that the causes of the failures were a stump that was too short and the loss of continuity between the proximal ulna and the TFCC and radioulnar ligament complex. Three patients were treated by insertion of an intercalary tricortical iliac crest bone graft into the site of the previous osteotomy and resection of the previous fusion of the distal ulna and radius, in a manner similar to a matched hemiresection. This procedure was augmented by soft tissue interposition. Fixation of the graft was achieved with a plate. The wrist was then splinted for 6 weeks. The investigators reported satisfaction in all 3 patients treated in this way, with full union on both sides of the graft. Two patients had their metalwork removed after union. All patients had returned to their previous occupation.[37]

Gonzalez del Pino and Fernandez[38] have described a technique for converting a failed Bowers hemiresection interposition to a Sauve-Kapanji procedure. They studied 3 patients who had Bowers procedure for severe degenerative changes within the DRUJ and had an intact TFCC. All the patients presented with severe DRUJ pain, decreased forearm rotation, and decreased grip strength. A 5/6 approach was made to the DRUJ. In all the patients, the interposed ECU tendon strip had atrophied and signs of radioulnar impingement were present. A segment of bone was resected from the ulna metaphysis to ensure a minimum gap of 10 mm. The resected segment was interposed between the distal ulna and the sigmoid notch, after denuding the surfaces with curettes and power burrs. The arthrodesis was fixed with lag screws. Pronator quadratus was pulled up to attach to the sheath of ECU. Stabilization was performed with either a palmar capsular flap or a distally based slip of FCU. A splint should be worn until union. The investigators reported that all patients were pain free, with unchanged or improved forearm rotation. At a minimum follow-up of 36 months (36–48 months, average 44 months), all patients had returned to previous work. In all patients, the DRUJ united solidly. The investigators advocate primary tenodesis of the stump with flexor carpi radialis to prevent more proximal stump impingement.[38]

If computed tomography demonstrates a flat or even, rounded, convex dorsal rim of the sigmoid notch and if it is thought that this is contributing to instability, the notch can be deepened by performing sigmoid notch osteoplasty as described by Wallwork and Bain.[39] This procedure is more likely to be indicated in situations in which there is instability of a distal ulna prosthesis and may be combined with soft tissue augmentation.

Distal Ulna Prosthetic Replacement

Alfred Swanson developed the first prosthesis for distal ulna replacement. This prosthesis, made of silicone, was intended as a spacer, and good outcomes were reported initially. However, the material properties of silicone did not allow longevity of the implant, and failure due to silicone synovitis was observed. McMurtry and colleagues[40] reported on 40 Swanson silicone ulnar head arthroplasties performed on 37 patients at a minimum of 12-months follow-up (12–48 months, average 29 months). Eight of the 40 procedures were performed for failed Darrach procedure. Satisfactory results were reported only in 37.5% of the patients in whom the Darrach procedure failed. Instability of the prosthesis was present in 56% of the unsatisfactory results. Fracture of the stem of the prosthesis was observed in radiographs of 29% of cases with rheumatoid

arthritis but not in those with failed Darrach procedure. Two cases of silicone synovitis were reported in this series. Bone resorption of the distal ulna was often seen, and it became worse with longer follow-up. This study prompted the investigators to abandon the procedure.

Herbert, encouraged by the early promise of the Swanson implant, developed a prosthesis with a titanium stem and zirconium oxide ceramic head (Herbert Ulnar Head Prosthesis, Gebrüder Martin GmbH & Co KG, Tuttlingen, Germany). This is an uncemented implant with a near spherical head. The distal surface is flat in this prosthesis. There are no holes for attachment of soft tissues. The implant is suitable for use in primary DRUJ arthrosis and for the management of failed DRUJ surgery. Herbert and van Schoonhoven[41] reported good long-term outcomes with low rates of loosening observed radiologically. Recurrent instability, ulnar impaction, stem loosening, periprosthetic fracture, and recurrent pain because of ectopic calcification or sigmoid erosion have been recorded.[41] The stability of this implant depends on strong capsular repair to the dorsal rim of the radius through bone tunnels, to allow scar formation around the head and neck of the implant.

The long-term outcome of salvage of failed resection arthroplasties using the Herbert Ulnar Head Prosthesis has been reported in a multicenter study of 16 of 23 patients followed up for a minimum of 97 months (97–154 months, average 133 months). All patients had a stable DRUJ and none required further surgery. Pain scores were significantly reduced from the preoperative scores, and there were no radiological signs of loosening.

For a failed Sauve-Kapanji procedure, a modified implant with a spherical head is available.[42] The procedure requires removal of all previous hardware and reaming of a socket in the fused ulna head to accommodate two-thirds of the spherical prosthetic head. Transverse distal radial osteotomy with preservation of the radial cortex may be required to help in positioning of the prosthesis into the socket, avoiding fracture of the ulna head. Fernandez and colleagues[42] presented the results for the use of this prosthesis in 10 patients at a minimum of 8-months follow-up (8–74 months, average 31 months). Six patients were pain free, and 4 had residual mild pain. Range of movement improved in 7 patients and worsened in 2. Among the 10 patients, 9 returned to their previous occupation. The prosthesis was stable in all patients. There were 2 fractures of the previous radioulnar arthrodesis, which were treated with screw fixation.[42] An alternative procedure has been used with success. This procedure requires the removal of the screw holding the ulna head to the radius and removing one-third to half of the head, with the osteotomy being in the coronal plane; the cancellous bone is then removed from the remaining part of the head, thus forming an exaggerated sigmoid notch. A prosthesis is then inserted into the prepared proximal ulna stump, and an appropriate neck length of the implant is chosen to allow the head of the prosthesis to engage within the exaggerated sigmoid notch (**Fig. 3**).

For the failed hemiresection interposition arthroplasty, a TFCC-preserving implant is available. The Eclypse implant (Bioprofile, Grenoble, France) consists of a semicylindrical pyrocarbon spacer, shaped to mimic the joint surface of the distal ulna.[43] This spacer is held in place by a titanium stem implanted into the distal ulna that has a peg over which the spacer is placed. The spacer can rotate slightly around the peg, and proximal-distal translation is possible. Short-term follow-up in 3 cases reported by the investigators, suggest encouraging outcomes at an average of less than 1 year.

The First Choice DRUJ system developed by Ascension Orthopedics Inc, Austin, TX, USA,[44] provides a resurfacing option intended for use in primary DRUJ procedures, but which may be suitable in some cases of salvage for failed matched hemiresection, in which the ulna styloid and TFCC attachments have been preserved. For the failed Darrach or Sauve-Kapanji procedure, Ascension Orthopedics Inc provides a modular ulnar head for restoration of ulnar head offset. This prosthesis has no holes for attachment of soft tissues and therefore relies on the joint capsule, ECU tendon, and scar tissue to maintain stability. No long-term follow-up data are available for this implant.

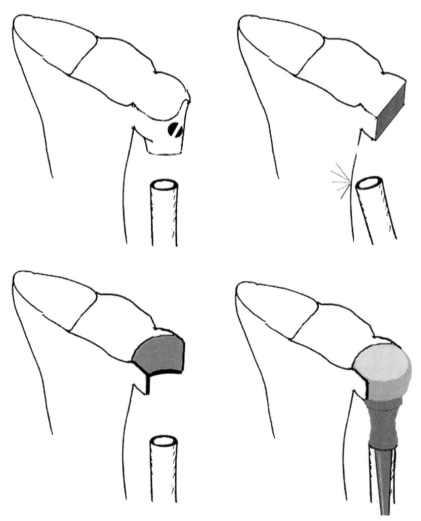

Fig. 3. Salvage of the failed Sauve-Kapanji procedure with head-in-head distal ulna replacement.

The Avanta uHead prosthesis (Small Bone Innovations Inc, Morrisville, PA, USA) is a modular distal ulnar replacement, which can be implanted cementless or cemented if the bone quality or fit is poor. This prosthesis has an advantage over the First Choice DRUJ system, because it has drill holes in the head that allow fixation of the soft tissue stabilizers, the TFCC, ECU subsheath, and dorsal capsule (**Fig. 4**). Berger and Cooney[33] reported on 22 patients who were followed up for 2 years. Two patients required additional soft tissue stabilization with the Linscheid-Hui ligament reconstruction at the initial surgery. The investigators reported good to excellent results in 18 of 22 patients. Two patients were revised for stem loosening, and 1 for implant malpositioning. One patient had persistent instability but had not undergone any further surgery.[33] The investigators noted that bone resorption just proximal to the implant collar is common, and it usually stabilizes at an average of 3 mm, at 6 months after implantation. A further report of 19 patients presumably includes the patients in whom the same prosthesis has been implanted.[45]

Scheker and colleagues[46] have devised a semi-constrained modular implant that consists of a stainless steel plate with a socket at the end, which is attached to the distal radius by a peg at the level of the socket. This plate articulates with a sphere made from ultra-high-molecular-weight polyethylene that is held in place by an ulna-stemmed highly polished peg, fitting in to a hole in the sphere, and a socket cover, enveloping the sphere, and attaches to the radial plate. The investigators' initial experience using this prosthesis in 23 patients with an average follow-up of 15 months was good, with all patients reporting complete pain relief, but the authors have concerns about the longevity of this prosthesis because of the significant forces transferred to the implant-radius interface.

The authors think that replacement of the ulna head to reconstruct the condylar cam of the distal ulna is essential to restore forearm stability in cases of failed DRUJ surgery. An algorithm is proposed to guide reconstruction in this situation (**Fig. 5**). In cases in which this reconstruction fails, with instability of the prosthesis, persistent pain, infection, or prosthesis loosening, salvage options are available. At the authors' institution the one-bone forearm procedure is preferred over wide excision of the ulna because the results are more predictable.

Wide Excision of Ulna

With the current understanding of the kinematics of the forearm, it seems counterintuitive to treat failed distal ulna surgery with resection of more of the ulna; indeed Bell and colleagues[22] described this as irrational as far back as 1985. It was anticipated that this procedure would fail because of radioulnar instability, more proximal stump impingement, dorsal translation of the stump on pronation, and ulnar translation of the carpus.[47] Occasionally, however, the surgeon may be left with few other options. The largest report of the outcome of wide distal ulna excision was a multicenter retrospective review of 12 patients followed up for a minimum of 6 months (6–62 months, average 22 months). Nine patients underwent wide distal ulnar excisions to treat failed DRUJ surgery (2 DRUJ surgeries were performed by matched hemiresection, 2 by Darrach procedure, 1 by debridement for osteomyelitis, 2 by Sauve-Kapanji procedures, and 2 by soft tissue stabilizations of the DRUJ). These 9 patients had undergone an average of 3 previous surgical procedures, whereas the other 3 patients had undergone radiocarpal fusion for degenerative disease. The average ulna resection in this series was 8 cm (33% of the ulna length), with a range from 6 to 11 cm (25%–50%). In all the cases for failed DRUJ surgery, subperiosteal resection was performed.

The investigators reported satisfactory clinical, radiographic, and functional outcomes in 7 of 9 patients, with forearm rotation averaging 89% of the opposite side. The 2 patients with failed results had immediate failure demonstrated by pain from the remaining ulna stump. The cause for failure in these 2 cases was attributed to incompetence of the central band of the interosseous membrane. The investigators recommended that the safe

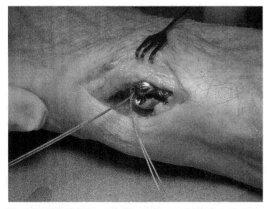

Fig. 4. Distal ulna replacement with the Avanta uHead prosthesis allows suturing of the TFCC to the prosthesis.

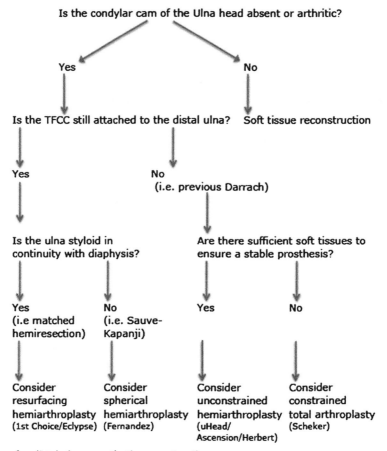

Fig. 5. Algorithm for distal ulnar prosthetic reconstruction.

zone for resection is between 25% and 45% of the ulna length and that a longitudinal instability of the forearm (Essex-Lopresti lesion) is a contraindication.[48]

The One-Bone Forearm Procedure

The one-bone forearm procedure was first described by Hey Groves[49] in 1921. Pain and instability, failed reconstructive surgery, or significant irreparable bone loss are the indications for this procedure.[50] The forearm should be fused between neutral rotation and pronation; however, the authors prefer a position of slight pronation. Peterson and colleagues[51] described 2 groups of patients in whom a one-bone forearm procedure may be indicated: (1) patients with posttraumatic instability and (2) patients with instability after oncological resection or due to congenital deformity. The investigators reported that less-favorable outcomes occur in

association with traumatic pathology, 2 or more previous reconstructive procedures, coexisting severe nerve injury, and previous episodes of infection. In this series, the rate of nonunion was 32%. Allende and Allende[52] reported on 7 patients treated for severe forearm trauma by the one-bone forearm procedure. The investigators used a combination of intramedullary and external fixations and percutaneous screw fixation to avoid significant soft tissue dissection. Autologous iliac crest bone graft was used in arthrodesis in all cases. Patients were followed up for a minimum of 6 years (6–16 years, average 9.7 years). All patients had a stable and pain-free forearm. The arthrodesis had healed within 14 weeks in all patients. Four patients had an excellent result, whereas 3 had good results. All patients returned to their previous occupation. Grip strength was 86% of the opposite side on average.[52] It remains unclear whether significant intraarticular ulnohumeral pathologic conditions

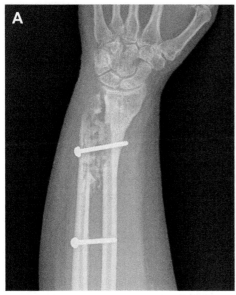 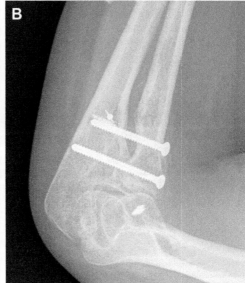

Fig. 6. Radiographs demonstrating osteotomy (*A*) and fixation for the one-bone forearm procedure (*B*).

or instability are contraindications to the one-bone forearm procedure.[51]

The authors' preferred method for creation of a one-bone forearm is to aim to create a proximal and distal radioulnar synostosis. This creation can be achieved by performing a coronal osteotomy through the distal ulna and opening it up like a book toward the radius. A matched osteotomy is performed on the ulna cortex of the radius and then is opened in the opposite direction to face the previous ulna osteotomy. Decortication of bone can be performed at the proximal radioulnar joint too. Fixation is achieved with two 3.5-mm cortical screws passed between the radius and ulna at each arthrodesis site (**Fig. 6**). Autologous bone graft from the iliac crest can also be used. This technique is the treatment of choice in the authors' institution for the failed distal ulna prosthetic reconstruction, but the expectations from the patient must be realistic because this procedure does not restore normal function. The authors' experience in this group of patients, who have undergone multiple previous operations and suffered a long period of pain, has been that the relief of pain symptoms is sufficient to ensure satisfaction.

SUMMARY

It is the authors' practice to attempt to reconstruct the distal ulna in the patient with failed primary DRUJ surgery. Consideration is given to what native restraints are preserved in preoperative assessment and planning. Satisfactory results can be achieved if attention is given to both

osseous and soft tissue restraint. If these procedures fail, the authors consider that a one-bone forearm procedure, with arthrodesis proximally and distally in the forearm, is most likely to give a satisfactory result with relief of pain but at the expense of limited function.

REFERENCES

1. Hagert CG. The distal radioulnar joint in relation to the whole forearm. Clin Orthop Relat Res 1992; 275:56.
2. af Ekenstam F. Anatomy of the distal radioulnar joint. Clin Orthop Relat Res 1992;275:14.
3. De Smet L, Fabry G. Orientation of the sigmoid notch of the distal radius: determination of different types of the distal radioulnar joint. Acta Orthop Belg 1993;59:269.
4. Tolat AR, Stanley JK, Trail IA. A cadaveric study of the anatomy and stability of the distal radioulnar joint in the coronal and transverse planes. J Hand Surg Br 1996;21:587.
5. Forstner H. [Morphology of the distal radio-ulnar joint. Surgical orthopedic consequences]. Handchir Mikrochir Plast Chir 1990;22:296 [in German].
6. Kauer JM. The distal radioulnar joint. Anatomic and functional considerations. Clin Orthop Relat Res 1992;275:37.
7. Bain GI, Pugh DM, MacDermid JC, et al. Matched hemiresection interposition arthroplasty of the distal radioulnar joint. J Hand Surg Am 1995;20:944.
8. Ray RD, Johnson RJ, Jameson RM. Rotation of the forearm; an experimental study of pronation and supination. J Bone Joint Surg Am 1951;33:993.

9. Stuart PR, Berger RA, Linscheid RL, et al. The dorsopalmar stability of the distal radioulnar joint. J Hand Surg Am 2000;25:689.

10. Palmer AK, Werner FW. Biomechanics of the distal radioulnar joint. Clin Orthop Relat Res 1984;187:26.

11. Field J, Majkowski RJ, Leslie IJ. Poor results of Darrach's procedure after wrist injuries. J Bone Joint Surg Br 1993;75:53.

12. Nolan WB 3rd, Eaton RG. A Darrach procedure for distal ulnar pathology derangements. Clin Orthop Relat Res 1992;275:85.

13. Tulipan DJ, Eaton RG, Eberhart RE. The Darrach procedure defended: technique redefined and long-term follow-up. J Hand Surg Am 1991;16:438.

14. Mikić ZD, Helal B. The value of the Darrach procedure in the surgical treatment of rheumatoid arthritis. Clin Orthop Relat Res 1977;127:175.

15. George MS, Kiefhaber TR, Stern PJ. The Sauve-Kapandji procedure and the Darrach procedure for distal radio-ulnar joint dysfunction after Colles' fracture. J Hand Surg Br 2004;29:608.

16. DiBenedetto MR, Lubbers LM, Coleman CR. Long-term results of the minimal resection Darrach procedure. J Hand Surg Am 1991;16:445.

17. Sotereanos DG, Leit ME. A modified Darrach procedure for treatment of the painful distal radioulnar joint. Clin Orthop Relat Res 1996;325:140.

18. Tsai TM, Shimizu H, Adkins P. A modified extensor carpi ulnaris tenodesis with the Darrach procedure. J Hand Surg Am 1993;18:697.

19. Taleisnik J. The Sauve-Kapandji procedure. Clin Orthop Relat Res 1992;275:110.

20. Bieber EJ, Linscheid RL, Dobyns JH, et al. Failed distal ulna resections. J Hand Surg Am 1988;13:193.

21. McKee MD, Richards RR. Dynamic radio-ulnar convergence after the Darrach procedure. J Bone Joint Surg Br 1996;78:413.

22. Bell MJ, Hill RJ, McMurtry RY. Ulnar impingement syndrome. J Bone Joint Surg Br 1985;67:126.

23. Sauerbier M, Hahn ME, Fujita M, et al. Analysis of dynamic distal radioulnar convergence after ulnar head resection and endoprosthesis implantation. J Hand Surg Am 2002;27:425.

24. Sauerbier M, Fujita M, Hahn ME, et al. The dynamic radioulnar convergence of the Darrach procedure and the ulnar head hemiresection interposition arthroplasty: a biomechanical study. J Hand Surg Br 2002;27:307.

25. Lees VC, Scheker LR. The radiological demonstration of dynamic ulnar impingement. J Hand Surg Br 1997;22:448–50.

26. Breen TF, Jupiter JB. Extensor carpi ulnaris and flexor carpi ulnaris tenodesis of the unstable distal ulna. J Hand Surg Am 1989;14:612.

27. Tsai TM, Stilwell JH. Repair of chronic subluxation of the distal radioulnar joint (ulnar dorsal) using flexor carpi ulnaris tendon. J Hand Surg Br 1984;9:289.

28. Johnson RK. Stabilization of the distal ulna by transfer of the pronator quadratus origin. Clin Orthop Relat Res 1992;275:130.

29. Ruby LK, Ferenz CC, Dell PC. The pronator quadratus interposition transfer: an adjunct to resection arthroplasty of the distal radioulnar joint. J Hand Surg Am 1996;21:60.

30. Sauerbier M, Berger RA, Fujita M, et al. Radioulnar convergence after distal ulnar resection: mechanical performance of two commonly used soft tissue stabilizing procedures. Acta Orthop Scand 2003;74:420.

31. Shah M, Klimisch J. Treatment of failed Darrach procedure including the brachioradialis sling. Curr Opin Orthop 2003;14:222.

32. Kleinman WB, Greenberg JA. Salvage of the failed Darrach procedure. J Hand Surg Am 1995;20:951.

33. Berger RA, Cooney WP 3rd. Use of an ulnar head endoprosthesis for treatment of an unstable distal ulnar resection: review of mechanics, indications, and surgical technique. Hand Clin 2005;21:603.

34. Sotereanos DG, Gobel F, Vardakas DG, et al. An allograft salvage technique for failure of the Darrach procedure: a report of four cases. J Hand Surg Br 2002;27:317.

35. Watson HK, Brown RE. Ulnar impingement syndrome after Darrach procedure: treatment by advancement lengthening osteotomy of the ulna. J Hand Surg Am 1989;14:302.

36. Hove LM, Helland P. Salvage of failed resection of the distal ulna. Case report. Scand J Plast Reconstr Surg Hand Surg 1999;33:453.

37. Ross M, Thomas J, Couzens G, et al. Salvage of the unstable Sauve-Kapandji procedure: a new technique. Tech Hand Up Extrem Surg 2007;11:87.

38. Gonzalez del Pino J, Fernandez DL. Salvage procedure for failed Bowers' hemiresection interposition technique in the distal radioulnar joint. J Hand Surg Br 1998;23:749.

39. Wallwork NA, Bain GI. Sigmoid notch osteoplasty for chronic volar instability of the distal radioulnar joint: a case report. J Hand Surg Am 2001;26:454.

40. McMurtry RY, Paley D, Marks P, et al. A critical analysis of Swanson ulnar head replacement arthroplasty: rheumatoid versus nonrheumatoid. J Hand Surg Am 1990;15:224.

41. Herbert TJ, van Schoonhoven J. Ulnar head replacement. Tech Hand Up Extrem Surg 2007;11:98.

42. Fernandez DL, Joneschild ES, Abella DM. Treatment of failed Sauve-Kapandji procedures with a spherical ulnar head prosthesis. Clin Orthop Relat Res 2006;445:100.

43. Garcia-Elias M. Eclypse: partial ulnar head replacement for the isolated distal radio-ulnar joint arthrosis. Tech Hand Up Extrem Surg 2007;11:121.

44. Kopylov P, Tagil M. Distal radioulnar joint replacement. Tech Hand Up Extrem Surg 2007;11:109.

45. Willis AA, Berger RA, Cooney WP 3rd. Arthroplasty of the distal radioulnar joint using a new ulnar head endoprosthesis: preliminary report. J Hand Surg Am 2007;32:177.

46. Scheker LR, Babb BA, Killion PE. Distal ulnar prosthetic replacement. Orthop Clin North Am 2001;32:365.

47. Thirupathi RG, Vuletin JC, Wadwa R, et al. Desmoplastic fibroma of the ulna. A case report. Clin Orthop Relat Res 1983;179:231.

48. Wolfe SW, Mih AD, Hotchkiss RN, et al. Wide excision of the distal ulna: a multicenter case study. J Hand Surg Am 1998;23:222.

49. Hey Groves EW. On modern methods of treating fractures. 2nd edition. Bristol (England): John Wright and Sons; 1921.

50. Murray RA. The one-bone forearm: a reconstructive procedure. J Bone Joint Surg Am 1955;37:366.

51. Peterson CA 2nd, Maki S, Wood MB. Clinical results of the one-bone forearm. J Hand Surg Am 1995;20:609.

52. Allende C, Allende BT. Posttraumatic one-bone forearm reconstruction. A report of seven cases. J Bone Joint Surg Am 2004;86:364.

Management of Injuries to the Interosseous Membrane

Julie E. Adams, MD[a],*, Scott P. Steinmann, MD[b],
A. Lee Osterman, MD[c]

KEYWORDS

- Interosseous membrane • Forearm longitudinal instability
- Radioulnar instability • Essex-Lopresti injury
- Interosseous ligament

Peter Essex-Lopresti described 2 cases in a posthumously published article that details the injury that now bears his name; however, others described this condition before this report.[1,2] This injury results from axial forces to the forearm that disrupt the radial head, the central band of the interosseous membrane (IOM), and the distal radial ulnar joint (DRUJ) through the triangular fibrocartilage complex (TFCC).[3,4]

ANATOMY AND BIOMECHANICS

The IOM is a complex set of fibers originating from the radius and inserting on the ulna. The central band portion, a 1.1-cm wide band, is the major load-bearing portion of the IOM and plays a role in axial stability of the forearm. The fibers of the central band run obliquely from distal ulnar to proximal radial in a 21° orientation to the long axis of the forearm, originating at one-third of the length of the ulna and inserting at 60% of the length of the radius proximally (**Fig. 1**). Other portions of the IOM include a thin membranous portion, a proximal band, and a variable number of accessory bands.[5–9]

In the intact setting, the radial head plays a role as the primary stabilizer of the forearm to axial load

and to preserve axial stability. However, when the radial head is disrupted or surgically removed, the central band of the IOM and the TFCC assume a greater role than their usual status as secondary stabilizers of the forearm.[7,9] In the Essex-Lopresti lesion, an axial load to the forearm results in injury to the radial head along with the central band of the IOM and the TFCC complex.[3,4] If the radial head is excised, longitudinal instability of the forearm may occur in the acute setting. Alternatively, in the chronic setting, an incomplete IOM or unhealed injury is subjected to forces that cause gradual attenuation of the IOM and subsequent longitudinal instability. Sequelae of radioulnar instability include proximal migration of the radius and development of radiocapitellar pain and arthrosis, ulnar-sided wrist pain from ulnar impaction, and forearm discomfort.[3,10]

TREATMENT

Considerations for treatment are predicated on making the diagnosis. The true extent of injury is frequently underappreciated. In one series, 15 of 20 cases were diagnosed after a mean delay of about 8 years after injury (range, 1 month–26 years).[11] In another series, forearm instability was

This work was not supported by any funding source.
[a] Department of Orthopedic Surgery, University of Minnesota, 2450 Riverside Avenue, R200, Minneapolis, MN 55454, USA
[b] Department of Orthopedic Surgery, Mayo Clinic, 200 First Street South West, Rochester, MN 55905, USA
[c] Philadelphia Hand Center, Thomas Jefferson University, 700 South Henderson Road, Suite 200, King of Prussia, PA 19078, USA
* Corresponding author.
E-mail address: adams854@umn.edu

Hand Clin 26 (2010) 543–548
doi:10.1016/j.hcl.2010.05.003
0749-0712/10/$ – see front matter © 2010 Elsevier Inc. All rights reserved.

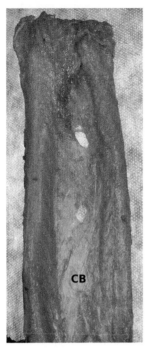

Fig. 1. Cadaveric specimen demonstrating fibers of the IOM. The central band (CB) is shown.

diagnosed at an average of 10 months (range, 2 month–12 years) after radial head excision.[12]

Attention is often focused on the obvious radial head fracture and elbow injury, whereas the injury to the forearm and ulnar wrist may be unrecognized. In one series of 106 referred Essex-Lopresti injuries, the complete diagnosis was made only 38% of the time.[12] The loss of continuity of the IOM, if untreated, results in the proximal migration of the radius and the sequelae of ulnar wrist pain and forearm and wrist weakness.[3] Alternatively, longitudinal forearm instability may occur after radial head resection in a chronic setting.[13] This instability may be because of an unhealed acute injury of the IOM or gradual attenuation of the ligament over time. The results are radiocapitellar impingement and ulnar impaction.[10,13] Some series suggest poorer outcomes in the setting of a delayed diagnosis.[11,14]

Treatment options are based on acuity of the injury (**Fig. 2**) and consideration of the wrist, forearm, and elbow.

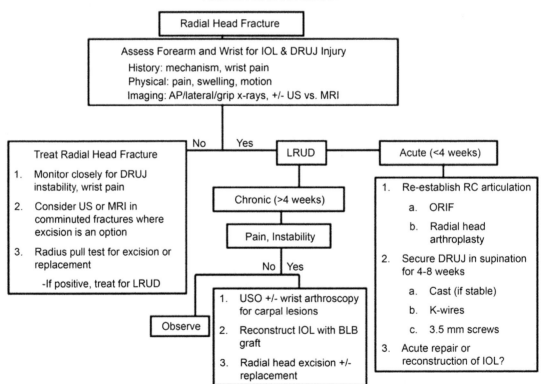

Fig. 2. Suggested treatment algorithm. AP, anteroposterior; BLB, bone ligament bone; IOL, interosseous ligament; LRUD, longitudinal radioulnar dissociation; MRI, magnetic resonance imaging; ORIF, open reduction and internal fixation; US, ultrasound; USO, ulnar shortening osteotomy. (*From* Marcotte AL, Osterman AL. Longitudinal radioulnar dissociation: identification and treatment of acute and chronic injuries. Hand Clin 2007;23(2):202, vi; with permission.)

Acute injuries (<1 month) are treated with fixation or replacement of the radial head to restore radiocapitellar force transmission and to prevent proximal migration of the radius. In delayed diagnosis, however, one should beware radial head replacement in the setting of established radiocapitellar changes. Placing a metallic radial head to articulate against damaged or arthritic capitellar cartilage may worsen elbow pain. Furthermore, although the radial head arthroplasty in the acute setting may function as a spacer to prevent migration, without healing of the IOM and TFCC, continued loads through the radiocapitellar joint in longitudinal instability may cause wear of the capitellar cartilage against the metallic head and radiocapitellar pain and arthrosis can develop.[5,14]

Excision of the radial head without stabilization of the longitudinal axis of the forearm is undesirable in longitudinal instability because without the restraint of the radial head, proximal migration of the radius occurs. However, radial head excision may be performed if stability of the forearm is restored, as with reconstruction of the IOM.[4,7,9,13–15]

At the forearm level, the goal is to restore longitudinal stability by stabilizing the forearm axis to allow healing of the IOM, reconstructing the IOM, or by substituting for the function of IOM.

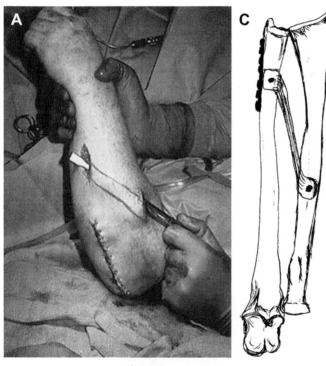

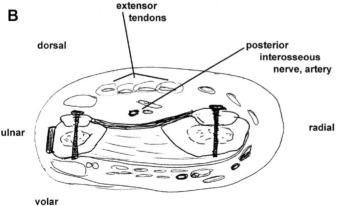

Fig. 3. (*A*) Intraoperative photograph depicting passage of the graft. A Kelly hemostat is passed from distal ulna to proximal radius at a 21° angle to the shaft to replicate the fibers of the central band. (*B*) Cross-sectional image showing placement of the graft. (*C*) Reconstruction. (*From* Adams JE, Culp RW, Osterman AL. Interosseous membrane reconstruction for the Essex-Lopresti injury. J Hand Surg Am 2010;35(1):134; with permission.)

In acute injuries, some investigators advocate stabilization of the forearm with splinting in supination or transfixion pinning with K wires or screws for a period to allow for intrinsic healing of the IOM, whereas others suggest that there is little healing capacity for the IOM.[7,16] Likewise, direct repair has been described,[17] although in Osterman and colleagues'[12] series of 10 acute explorations, most were midligament tears that were poorly amenable to repair and separated in vivo by the presence of tissue interposition and displacement of the forearm bones.[5] However, augmentation of the central band in acute tears by rerouting the pronator teres has been used with success. The pronator is left attached distally, while its proximal portion is elevated at the musculotendinous junction, rotated distally, and attached to the ulna to replicate the orientation of the central band fibers.[18]

Multiple techniques have been described using various tissues for reconstruction of the IOM, including tendon auto- or allografts, pronator teres, synthetic materials, or bone-tendon-bone graft.[5,9,14,16,18–22] One large series has shown success with the use of bone–patellar-tendon–bone autograft to reconstruct longitudinal radioulnar instability injuries in the chronic setting.[5,12,14]

Creation of a radioulnar synostosis is a salvage procedure, although the disadvantages are necessarily fixing the forearm in one permanent rotational position and, for indications of posttraumatic reconstruction, complications, including nonunion, are more likely than for those who have the procedure for other reasons.[23,24]

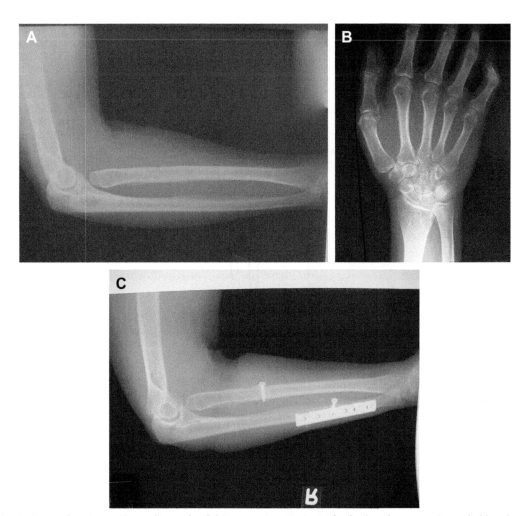

Fig. 4. Pre- and postoperative radiographs. (*A*) Forearm in a patient who had undergone prior radial head excision for a fracture. (*B*) She developed ulnar-positive variance because of chronic longitudinal instability of the forearm. (*C*) The patient underwent ulnar shortening osteotomy and IOM reconstruction with a bone–patellar-tendon–bone allograft.

In the acute wrist injury, the TFCC is repaired and stability of the DRUJ restored. In the chronic setting, ulnar impaction is addressed by a joint-leveling procedure and arthroscopic debridement of the TFCC. Ulnar shortening osteotomy alone may allow for recurrence of ulnar impaction if the forearm is not stabilized.[14,25]

One treatment algorithm proposed by one of the authors (ALO) has been used in a large series of chronic cases (see **Fig. 2**). The technique is described elsewhere.[5,12,14] Briefly, wrist arthroscopy is performed to evaluate ulnar impaction and to debride the TFCC. An ulnar shortening osteotomy addresses ulnar impaction. At the forearm level, a bone–patellar tendon graft is used to reconstruct the central band of the IOM. One bony end of the graft is secured to a bony trough created in the ulna at the ulnar insertion of the IOM with a 3.5-mm screw. The other end of the graft is then passed under the extensor tendons to the interval between the extensor carpi radialis longus and brachioradialis, to the radial insertion site, with care taken to avoid the superficial radial nerve. The graft is oriented to replicate the 21° orientation to the forearm axis and tensioned in semisupination before being secured to the radial trough via a second screw (**Figs. 3** and **4**). The outcomes after this technique have been described in a series of 46 patients with an average follow-up approaching 10 years. No patient had recurrent instability. Ninety-four percent described relief of wrist pain, and elbow discomfort was lessened. Grip strengths improved from 59% to 86% postoperatively.[12]

SUMMARY

Essex-Lopresti injuries are complex injuries involving the elbow, the forearm through the IOM, and the wrist. Treatment strategies are aimed at each of these areas.

REFERENCES

1. Brockman EP. Two cases of disability at the wrist following excision of the head of the radius. Proc R Soc Med 1931;24:904–5.
2. Curr JF, Coe WA. Dislocation of the inferior radio-ulnar joint. Br J Surg 1946;34:74–7.
3. Dodds SD, Yeh PC, Slade JF 3rd. Essex-Lopresti injuries. Hand Clin 2008;24(1):125–37.
4. Essex-Lopresti P. Fractures of the radial head with distal radio-ulnar dislocation; report of two cases. J Bone Joint Surg Br 1951;33B(2):244–7.
5. Adams JE, Culp RW, Osterman AL. Interosseous membrane reconstruction for the Essex-Lopresti injury. J Hand Surg Am 2010;35(1):129–36.
6. Green JB, Zelouf DS. Forearm instability. J Hand Surg Am 2009;34(5):953–61.
7. Hotchkiss RN, An KN, Sowa DT, et al. An anatomic and mechanical study of the interosseous membrane of the forearm: pathomechanics of proximal migration of the radius. J Hand Surg Am 1989;14(2 Pt 1):256–61.
8. Noda K, Goto A, Murase T, et al. Interosseous membrane of the forearm: an anatomical study of ligament attachment locations. J Hand Surg Am 2009;34(3):415–22.
9. Skahen JR 3rd, Palmer AK, Werner FW, et al. Reconstruction of the interosseous membrane of the forearm in cadavers. J Hand Surg Am 1997;22(6):986–94.
10. Shepard MF, Markolf KL, Dunbar AM. The effects of partial and total interosseous membrane transection on load sharing in the cadaver forearm. J Orthop Res 2001;19(4):587–92.
11. Trousdale RT, Amadio PC, Cooney WP, et al. Radioulnar dissociation. A review of twenty cases. J Bone Joint Surg Am 1992;74(10):1486–97.
12. Osterman AL, Warhold L, Culp RW, et al. Reconstruction of the interosseous membrane using a bone-ligament-bone graft. American Society for Surgery of the Hand 52nd Annual Meeting. Denver (CO), September 11–13, 1997.
13. Sowa DT, Hotchkiss RN, Weiland AJ. Symptomatic proximal translation of the radius following radial head resection. Clin Orthop Relat Res 1995;(317):106–13.
14. Marcotte AL, Osterman AL. Longitudinal radioulnar dissociation: identification and treatment of acute and chronic injuries. Hand Clin 2007;23(2):195–208, vi.
15. Smith AM, Urbanosky LR, Castle JA, et al. Radius pull test: predictor of longitudinal forearm instability. J Bone Joint Surg Am 2002;84(11):1970–6.
16. Ruch DS, Chang DS, Koman LA. Reconstruction of longitudinal stability of the forearm after disruption of interosseous ligament and radial head excision (Essex-Lopresti lesion). J South Orthop Assoc 1999;8(1):47–52.
17. Failla JM, Jacobson J, van Holsbeeck M. Ultrasound diagnosis and surgical pathology of the torn interosseous membrane in forearm fractures/dislocations. J Hand Surg Am 1999;24(2):257–66.
18. Chloros GD, Wiesler ER, Stabile KJ, et al. Reconstruction of Essex-Lopresti injury of the forearm: technical note. J Hand Surg Am 2008;33(1):124–30.
19. Pfaeffle HJ, Stabile KJ, Li ZM, et al. Reconstruction of the interosseous ligament restores normal forearm

compressive load transfer in cadavers. J Hand Surg Am 2005;30(2):319–25.

20. Pfaeffle HJ, Stabile KJ, Li ZM, et al. Reconstruction of the interosseous ligament unloads metallic radial head arthroplasty and the distal ulna in cadavers. J Hand Surg Am 2006;31(2):269–78.

21. Sellman DC, Seitz WH Jr, Postak PD, et al. Reconstructive strategies for radioulnar dissociation: a biomechanical study. J Orthop Trauma 1995;9(6):516–22.

22. Tomaino MM, Pfaeffle J, Stabile K, et al. Reconstruction of the interosseous ligament of the forearm reduces load on the radial head in cadavers. J Hand Surg Br 2003;28(3):267–70.

23. Chen F, Culp RW, Schneider LH, et al. Revision of the ununited one-bone forearm. J Hand Surg Am 1998;23(6):1091–6.

24. Peterson CA 2nd, Maki S, Wood MB. Clinical results of the one-bone forearm. J Hand Surg Am 1995; 20(4):609–18.

25. Morrey BF, Askew LJ, Chao EY. A biomechanical study of normal functional elbow motion. J Bone Joint Surg Am 1981;63(6):872–7.

Ulnar Impaction

Douglas M. Sammer, MD[a], Marco Rizzo, MD[b],*

KEYWORDS
- Ulnar impaction • Ulnocarpal impaction • Abutment
- Stylocarpal impaction

Ulnar impaction syndrome, also known as ulnocarpal impaction or ulnocarpal abutment, is a common source of ulnar-sided wrist pain. It is a degenerative condition that occurs secondary to excessive load across the ulnocarpal joint, resulting in a spectrum of pathologic changes and symptoms. It may occur in any wrist but is usually associated with positive ulnar variance, whether congenital or acquired. It may be seen after distal radius malunion, radial head excision, congenitally positive ulnar variance, premature physeal closure of the radius, or any condition that causes an increase in the relative length of the ulna. Mechanical abutment of the distal ulna with the carpus often results in pain and progressive deterioration of the triangular fibrocartilage complex (TFCC), as well as pathologic changes in the dome of the ulnar head, the ulnar corner of the lunate, the triquetrum, and the lunotriquetral interosseous ligament (LTIL). The diagnosis of ulnar impaction syndrome is made by clinical examination and is supported by radiographic studies. Surgery is indicated if nonoperative treatment fails. Although a number of alternatives exist, the 2 primary surgical options are ulnar-shortening osteotomy or partial resection of the distal dome of the ulna (wafer procedure). This article discusses the etiology of ulnar impaction syndrome, and its diagnosis and treatment.

BIOMECHANICS

In the ulnar neutral wrist, the ulnocarpal joint bears 18% of the load that crosses the wrist.[1] The TFCC plays a critical role in transferring this load from the carpus to the ulna. Excision of the TFCC decreases the load transmitted to the ulna by 67%, and the ulna bears only 6% of the total load across the wrist.[1] An inverse relationship between ulnar variance and TFCC thickness has been demonstrated[2]; therefore, a thick TFCC is present in wrists with congenital negative ulnar variance, allowing effective transfer of load from the carpus to the ulna. Although it is less common, ulnar impaction syndrome can occur in patients with neutral or negative ulnar variance.[3]

Forearm pronation and grip both result in a relative increase in ulnar length.[4–6] In ulnar neutral or negative wrists, this increase in relative length can be enough to create a dynamic positive ulnar variance. In the ulnar neutral wrist, this dynamic positive ulnar variance results in an increase in ulnocarpal load.[7,8] There is evidence that in some ulnar positive wrists, however, that the dynamic increase in relative ulnar length during pronation and grip leads to dorsal subluxation of the ulnar head, resulting in a decrease in ulnocarpal load.[8] In ulnar neutral or negative wrists, the phenomenon of dynamic positive ulnar variance with increased ulnocarpal load and the presence of a thicker TFCC explain the occurrence of ulnar impaction syndrome.

Increasing or decreasing the relative length of the ulna has been shown to cause significant changes in ulnocarpal load. In a study by Palmer and Werner,[1] increasing the length of the ulna by 2.5 mm resulted in an increase in ulnocarpal load to 42% of the total load across the wrist. On the other hand, decreasing the length of the ulna by 2.5 mm resulted in a decrease in ulnocarpal load to only 4% of the total load across the wrist. Resection of a wafer of the distal dome of the

[a] Division of Plastic Surgery, Washington University School of Medicine, Suite 1150, NW Tower, 660 South Euclid Avenue, Campus Box 8238, St Louis, MO 63110, USA
[b] Division of Hand Surgery, Department of Orthopedic Surgery, Mayo Clinic, 200 First Street SW, Rochester, MN 55905, USA
* Corresponding author.
E-mail address: rizzo.marco@mayo.edu

Hand Clin 26 (2010) 549–557
doi:10.1016/j.hcl.2010.05.011
0749-0712/10/$ – see front matter © 2010 Elsevier Inc. All rights reserved.

ulna has also been shown to decrease ulnocarpal load transmission, regardless of initial ulnar variance.[9,10] This decrease in ulnocarpal load is the rationale for the ulnar-shortening osteotomy and the wafer resection in the treatment of ulnar impaction syndrome.[11,12]

PRESENTATION

There is little information known about the demographics and natural history of ulnar impaction syndrome. Because ulnar variance tends to be more positive in Asian individuals than White, the incidence of idiopathic ulnar impaction syndrome may be higher in Asian populations.[13–19] Ulnar impaction syndrome is also more common in patients who have an acquired increase in ulnar variance, such as after a distal radius fracture malunion (**Fig. 1**). It is possible that with an increased tendency for distal radius fracture fixation, the incidence of acquired ulnar impaction syndrome will decrease.

The onset of symptoms is usually insidious and progressive. Patients complain of ulnar-sided wrist pain, and occasionally swelling and loss of wrist motion and forearm rotation. Symptoms are exacerbated by activities that involve forceful grip, pronation, and ulnar deviation. In cases of idiopathic ulnar impaction syndrome, patients do not typically report an acute traumatic event preceding the onset of symptoms. Not all cases of ulnar impaction are symptomatic. Although

ulnar impaction is presumably symptomatic in most cases, it is not unusual to see a patient with radiographic evidence of ulnar impaction, but who has minimal symptoms.

EXAMINATION AND DIAGNOSIS

The diagnosis of ulnar impaction syndrome is made on clinical grounds, and is supported by radiographic studies. A complete wrist examination should be performed to rule out other sources of pain such as pisotriquetral arthritis, distal radioulnar joint (DRUJ) arthrosis, extensor carpi ulnaris (ECU) subluxation or tendonitis, or neuritis of the dorsal cutaneous branch of the ulnar nerve. The ulnocarpal stress test was described by Nakamura and colleagues,[20] and involves placing the wrist in maximum ulnar deviation, axially loading the wrist, and passively rotating the forearm through supination to pronation (**Fig. 2**). A positive test is one in which the patient's typical pain is reproduced, and is suggestive of ulnar impaction syndrome. Although sensitive for ulnar impaction syndrome, a number of other pathologic processes can result in a positive ulnocarpal stress test, including LTIL injury, TFCC injury (without impaction), and isolated arthritis.[21] The patient will also have tenderness to palpation dorsally just distal to the head of the ulna, and ulnarly just volar to the styloid. The lunotriquetral interval may be tender. If the LTIL is involved, lunotriquetral provocative maneuvers such as the Regan shuck test and the Kleinman shear test may be positive. It is also important to examine the DRUJ for stability and pain, as this will affect

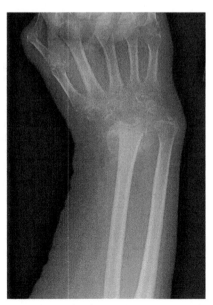

Fig. 1. PA radiograph of the right wrist 6 months after an untreated distal radius fracture. Note the severe positive ulnar variance.

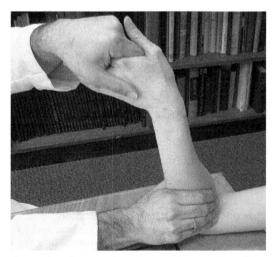

Fig. 2. The ulnocarpal stress test. The examiner places the wrist in maximum ulnar deviation, axially loads the wrist, and passively rotates the forearm from supination into pronation.

surgical decision making. It is also important to compare the affected wrist examination with the contralateral side.

IMAGING

As part of a standard wrist series, a neutral rotation posterior-anterior (PA) wrist radiograph should be obtained to determine ulnar variance. These are performed by imaging the wrist with the elbow flexed at 90 degrees and the forearm in neutral rotation. In addition, a pronated grip PA radiograph should be obtained to evaluate for dynamic positive ulnar variance.[5,6,22] All views should be evaluated for pathology that could lead to acquired positive ulnar variance, such as a malunited distal radius fracture or premature arrest of the distal radius physis. Comparison radiographs of the contralateral (unaffected) side are frequently helpful. Radiographs may demonstrate subchondral sclerosis or cystic changes at the dome of the ulna, the proximal ulnar corner of the lunate, or the proximal radial corner of the triquetrum.[22] In severe cases, changes consistent with frank degenerative arthritis, such as osteophyte formation, may be evident at the ulnocarpal joint. The PA radiograph should be examined for DRUJ arthritis, and the slope of the DRUJ should be noted in anticipation of possible ulnar-shortening osteotomy. The lateral radiograph should be evaluated for evidence of dorsal ulnar subluxation.[13] Although not usually necessary, if the diagnosis is unclear magnetic resonance imaging (MRI) provides detailed images of the structures involved, and is useful in detecting occult pathology.[22] In its earliest stages, the involved articular cartilage may develop fibrillation and chondromalacia, which can be detected on MRI. Bone hyperemia or edema, localized to the involved regions, may also be evident (**Fig. 3**).[22,23] Subtle subchondral sclerosis or cystic changes are also detectable by MRI. MRI, and in particular MR arthrography, is useful for evaluating the integrity of the TFCC and the LTIL.[24] When the diagnosis is in question, MRI is especially useful for evaluating other possible sources of ulnar-sided wrist pain.

PALMER CLASSIFICATION

The Palmer classification provides a scheme for categorizing acute and chronic TFCC injuries according to the location and severity of pathology seen on arthroscopy.[25] Class II conditions (IIA through IIE) are degenerative, as opposed to acute TFCC injuries, and represent a spectrum of increasing severity of pathology

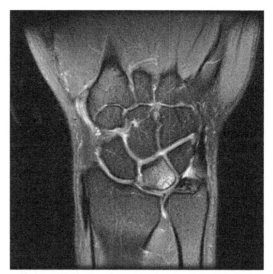

Fig. 3. A coronal MRI demonstrating edema changes in the lunate consistent with ulnocarpal impaction.

secondary to ulnar impaction syndrome (**Table 1**). It should be noted that Class IA injuries, which are acute traumatic central disk perforations, are difficult to differentiate from degenerative perforations secondary to ulnar impaction syndrome.[26]

TREATMENT

Nonoperative treatment should be provided initially, particularly in cases of idiopathic ulnar impaction syndrome. This should include 6 to 12 weeks of rest or immobilization, activity modification, nonsteroidal anti-inflammatory drugs, or local corticosteroids. If these modalities fail to

Table 1	
The Palmer classification of TFCC degenerative conditions (Class II lesions)	
Classification	**Description**
IIA	TFCC wear
IIB	TFCC wear + chondromalacia
IIC	TFCC perforation + chondromalacia
IID	TFCC perforation + chondromalacia + LTIL perforation
IIE	TFCC perforation + chondromalacia + LTIL perforation + arthritis

Abbreviations: LTIL, lunotriquetral interosseous ligament; TFCC, triangular fibrocartilage complex.

adequately treat symptoms, surgical intervention is indicated.

The goal of surgery for ulnar impaction syndrome is to decrease the length of the ulna relative to the radius, thereby diminishing the amount of load that crosses the ulnocarpal joint. The 2 primary options for accomplishing this goal are the ulnar-shortening osteotomy and the wafer procedure, both of which have been shown to decrease load across the ulnocarpal joint.[1,9–12,27] Although less well studied, a number of ulnar head excisional osteotomies have been described, all of which effectively shorten the ulnar head while preserving the domal cartilage.[28–30] Depending on severity and symptoms, the presence of coexisting DRUJ arthritis should lead to consideration of procedures that address pathology of both the DRUJ and the ulnar impaction syndrome. Although not the focus of this article, these include endoprosthetic ulnar head arthroplasty, Bowers' hemiresection interposition technique, matched distal ulna resection, the Darrach procedure, and the Sauve-Kapandji procedure.[31–34] Finally, in cases of acquired positive ulnar variance, the surgeon should consider correcting the underlying problem in the radius, as opposed to shortening the ulna.

Ulnar-Shortening Osteotomy

The ulnar-shortening osteotomy was first described by Milch[27] in 1941 (**Fig. 4**). It remains the gold standard against which other surgeries for ulnar impaction syndrome are compared. Although both ulnar-shortening osteotomy and the wafer procedure reduce ulnocarpal load and effectively treat the symptoms of ulnar impaction, there are some situations in which ulnar-shortening osteotomy should be preferred over the wafer procedure. In a wrist with both positive ulnar variance and a prominent ulnar styloid, resulting in ulnocarpal and stylocarpal impaction, an ulnar-shortening osteotomy should be performed because the wafer procedure will not address the stylocarpal impaction.[26,35] Another situation in which the ulnar-shortening osteotomy is advantageous is that of the ulnar impaction syndrome with dorsal subluxation of the ulna. A recent study by Baek and colleagues[13] demonstrated that in addition to shortening the ulna, ulnar-shortening osteotomy also decreases subluxation of the distal ulna. The amount of shortening with a wafer procedure is limited to 2 to 3 mm. If more than 2 to 3 mm of shortening is required, an ulnar-shortening osteotomy should be performed. There is some belief that shortening the ulna stabilizes the entire ulnar

ligamentous complex, and is preferable in situations in which there is LTIL injury.

The osteotomy should be performed at the junction of the distal and middle third of the ulna. Typically, a transverse or oblique osteotomy is made, and fixation is achieved with a compression plate. An incision is made along the subcutaneous border of the ulna. The length of the incision is determined by the length of the plate, and the distal end of the incision should be 4 cm proximal to the ulnar styloid. Dissection is carried down between the ECU and the flexor carpi ulnaris (FCU). The periosteum is incised longitudinally, and elevated circumferentially to the interosseous membrane. The plate should provide 3 bicortical screws proximal and distal to the osteotomy, and should provide compression. Some plates allow placement of a lag screw through an oblique osteotomy as well. The plate should be contoured to the ulna before creating the osteotomy. In addition, because the distal ulna becomes mobile after osteotomy, one of the distal screw holes should be drilled before creating the osteotomy. It is also important to created a longitudinal score in the cortex at the site of the proposed osteotomy, to prevent inadvertent rotation of the ulna.[36] In ulnar positive wrists, the ulna should be shortened to 0 to –1 mm ulnar variance.[36] In patients with neutral or negative ulnar variance preoperatively, the amount of resection required correlates with the degree of dynamic positive ulnar variance that occurs during pronation and grip. Ulnar-shortening osteotomy has been demonstrated in biomechanical studies to increase peak pressure at the DRUJ.[37] The greater the ulnar shortening, the greater the peak pressure. This suggests that the minimum required amount of ulnar shortening necessary to treat the problem should be performed. The surgeon should be aware of the kerf of the blade being used, as this will affect the size of the osteotomy. Hardware systems that include osteotomy guides and compression plates designed specifically for precise shortening of the ulna are available. Postoperatively, a sugar-tong splint is applied. At 2 weeks it is removed. Patients are provided with an elbow-hinged long-arm splint or a Muenster-type splint, and wrist and forearm range of motion outside of the splint is begun. Union is expected within 3 months.

Results after ulnar-shortening osteotomy are good and predictable, with improved Mayo Wrist scores, Disabilities of Arm, Shoulder and Hand scores, range of motion, grip strength, pain, and high satisfaction rates demonstrated in multiple studies.[13,38–41] The most common complications after an ulnar-shortening osteotomy include delayed union or nonunion, and hardware-related

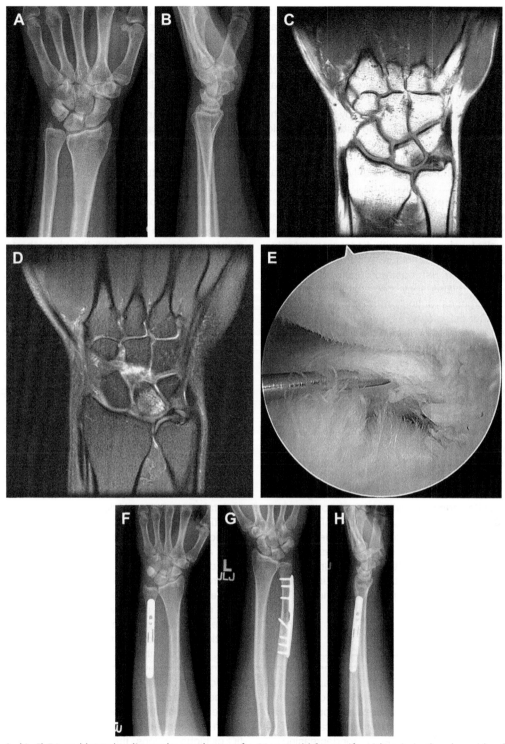

Fig. 4. (*A, B*) PA and lateral radiographs are shown of a 44-year-old farm wife with pain in the ulnar side of her left wrist. (*C, D*) T1- and T2-weighted coronal MRI shows typical changes within the lunate suggesting impaction. (*E*) A photograph taken during arthroscopy demonstrates a large central TFCC tear through which the probe is inserted. Note the chondromalacia of the articular surface of the lunate as well as on the surface of the ulnar head. (*F*) PA radiograph following the ulnar-shortening osteotomy is shown and demonstrates appropriate correction of the ulnar variance. (*G, H*) Final radiographs following osteotomy after healing of the ulna are shown.

problems. The nonunion rate is about 5%, but can be exacerbated by a number of factors.[21] Cigarette smoking increases the nonunion and delayed union rate after ulnar-shortening osteotomy, increasing the mean union time from 4 months to 7 months.[42] Smoking is therefore a relative contraindication to ulnar-shortening osteotomy. Delayed or nonunion can also be affected by surgical technique. Copious irrigation during osteotomy should be used to prevent thermal injury to the osteocytes. The periosteum should be carefully preserved during osteotomy. Only as much elevation as is required should be performed. Good compression is essential. Rayhack and colleagues suggested that an oblique osteotomy may improve union time, although other studies show equivalent union times with transverse osteotomies and careful technique.[13,43] Hardware palpability or pain is common, although newer low-profile plates may decrease this problem. Some surgeons routinely remove the plate 1 to 2 years after osteotomy, although this is not necessary in all patients.[21] Placing the plate on the volar, as opposed to dorsal or ulnar border of the ulna, should also reduce the need for later hardware removal. Furthermore, the volar surface of the ulna is often the flattest and widest.[40] Ulnar shortening should be avoided in patients with DRUJ arthritis, and in patients with a reverse oblique DRUJ slope. In this situation, significant shortening of the ulna may result in abnormal contact between the seat of the ulna and the proximal rim of the sigmoid notch.

It should be noted that ulnar-shortening osteotomy is often combined with wrist arthroscopy (see **Fig. 3**). This permits direct evaluation of the TFCC, LTIL, and articular surfaces. It allows debridement of the TFCC perforation or tear, if present. Cartilage flaps on the lunate or triquetrum articular surface can be resected. If LTIL injury is diagnosed, debridement is performed and the joint can be pinned.[36]

The Wafer Procedure

The wafer procedure (partial distal ulnar resection) was described by Feldon in 1992,[11,12] and involves resection of a thin wafer of the dome of the ulnar head (**Fig. 5**). Initially described as an open procedure, it can be performed arthroscopically as well. The wafer procedure is effective for decreasing ulnocarpal load and has some advantages over ulnar-shortening osteotomy. Constantine and colleagues[44] compared the clinical outcomes after ulnar-shortening osteotomy and wafer procedure. They found similar results in terms of pain relief and wrist function after both surgeries; however,

the ulnar-shortening osteotomy group required more revision operations for painful hardware, and delayed union occurred in some patients. Similar findings have been reported by other investigators.[45] The primary advantage of the wafer procedure is the lack of hardware-related complications, and the avoidance of delayed union or nonunion that can be seen with ulnar-shortening osteotomies. It can also be performed in wrists that have a reverse oblique slope of the DRUJ (see **Fig. 5A**). As noted previously, drawbacks to the wafer procedure include the 2- to 3-mm limit for ulnar resection and the fact that it does not address stylocarpal impaction (if present). Furthermore, it does not improve dorsal subluxation of the ulna, and it does not tighten the ulnocarpal ligamentous complex, as does the ulnar-shortening osteotomy. However, in most circumstances it can be an effective treatment for ulnar impaction syndrome, and avoids the hardware complications, delayed healing time, and repeat surgeries that can occur with ulnar-shortening osteotomy.

The open wafer procedure involves a longitudinal incision centered over the DRUJ. The extensor retinaculum is incised along the course of the extensor digiti quinti, which is retracted to the side. The joint capsule is then incised longitudinally, and then ulnarly across the dome of the ulna just proximal to the TFCC. Care must be taken to preserve the TFCC distally. Subperiosteal reflection in an ulnarward direction allows visualization of the ulnar head and the base of the styloid. The distal 2 to 3 mm of the ulnar dome is removed with a sagittal saw. It is important to protect and maintain the palmar and dorsal radioulnar ligament insertion at the fovea and at the base of the ulnar styloid. The TFCC is debrided from the undersurface. A layered closure is performed. The patient is placed in a sugar-tong splint, which is converted to a removable wrist cock-up brace at 2 weeks. Active motion is allowed time, but full activity does not resume until 8 weeks postoperatively.

The arthroscopic wafer procedure involves sufficient resection of the dome of the ulnar head, using an arthroscopic burr, such that the impaction is relieved. Initially, the TFCC is debrided with a shaver to a smooth, stable edge. Chondromalacia of the lunate surface can also be treated with the shaver. After the TFCC perforation is debrided in patients with Palmer class IIC or higher lesions, the dome of the ulna is accessed through the perforation. Typically 2 to 3 mm of ulnar head removal is sufficient; however, in cases of significant ulnar positive variance, more resection would be necessary. Care must be taken to excise the ulnar head area of impaction entirely. Adequate exposure for this can be

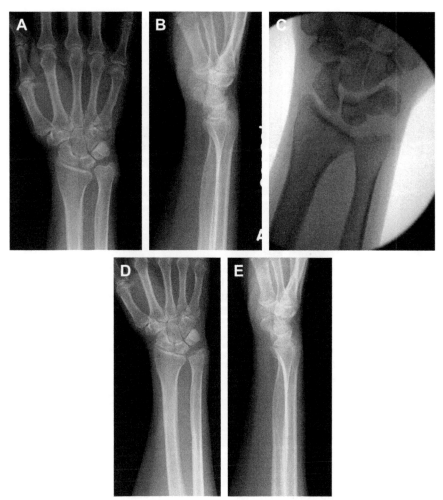

Fig. 5. (*A, B*) PA and lateral radiographs of a 52-year-old woman with ulnocarpal impaction. Note the reverse obliquity of the sigmoid notch. In addition, the bony changes of the ulnar side of the lunate consistent with ulnocarpal impaction can be seen on the PA view. (*C*) Intraoperative fluoroscopy confirms the appropriate amount of ulnar head is removed. Debridement and resection of the cartilage and subchondral bone down to the softer cancellous bone are usually necessary to alleviate the impaction. (*D, E*) Final PA and lateral films following the wafer procedure.

performed by pronating and supinating the forearm during the wafer procedure. This will reveal areas of the head that may need further resection. In addition, the use of intraoperative fluoroscopy will confirm that an appropriate amount of ulnar head has been removed (see **Fig. 5**C). Although some would advocate preserving the TFCC and converting to an open wafer procedure in patients with class IIA or IIB lesions, in which a TFCC perforation is not present, Tomaino and Elfar[26] report good results in these patients by resection of the central articular disk, followed by wafer resection. They note that resection of the central disk may contribute to unloading the joint, and also treats the fibrillation on the innervated undersurface of the TFCC.

Stylocarpal Impaction

A variant of ulnar impaction syndrome is that of stylocarpal impaction (**Fig. 6**). Differentiating this from ulnar impaction is important, as a wafer procedure would be an ineffective treatment for stylocarpal impaction. If ulnocarpal impaction and stylocarpal impaction are both present, an ulnar-shortening osteotomy should be performed. Tomaino and colleagues[35] reported a series of 5 patients who were treated for stylocarpal impaction. All underwent arthroscopy to rule out concomitant ulnar impaction syndrome. An ulnar styloid resection was performed at its base just distal to the TFCC insertion, with good results. All patients in this series had negative ulnar variance ranging from −3 to −7 mm, and had styloid

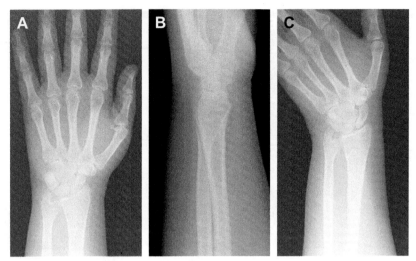

Fig. 6. (*A, B*) PA and lateral views of a 32-year-old woman with a large ulnar styloid and stylocarpal impaction. Note the negative ulnar variance of the ulna, which has been shown to be associated with stylocarpal impaction. (*C*) An ulnar deviation view nicely demonstrates impaction of the carpus on the prominent ulnar styloid.

processes that were greater than the normal length of 3 to 6 mm. Stylocarpal impaction occurs more commonly in wrists with negative ulnar variance, in which the styloid has excessive length.[35]

SUMMARY

Ulnar impaction syndrome is a common source of ulnar-sided wrist pain. It is most common in ulnar positive wrists, whether congenital or acquired, but can occur in ulnar neutral or negative wrists. Therefore, patients should be evaluated for dynamic positive ulnar variance. If the diagnosis is unclear, MRI is the most useful imaging modality. The ulnocarpal stress test should reproduce the patient's symptoms, and other sources of pain should be ruled out. Treatment requires decreasing the length of the ulna relative to the radius. In cases of acquired positive ulnar variance, treatment of the underlying cause in the radius should be considered, such as in distal radius malunion. In idiopathic ulnar impaction syndrome, the mainstays of surgical treatment are the ulnar-shortening osteotomy and the wafer procedure. Both operations are reliable in treating ulnar impaction syndrome. But because each operation has unique advantages and disadvantages, neither is ideal in every clinical situation and decision making must be individualized.

REFERENCES

1. Palmer AK, Werner FW. Biomechanics of the distal radioulnar joint. Clin Orthop Relat Res 1984;187: 26–35.

2. Palmer AK, Glisson RR, Werner FW. Relationship between ulnar variance and triangular fibrocartilage complex thickness. J Hand Surg Am 1984;9(5):681–2.

3. Tomaino MM. Ulnar impaction syndrome in the ulnar negative and neutral wrist. Diagnosis and pathoanatomy. J Hand Surg Br 1998;23(6):754–7.

4. Friedman SL, Palmer AK, Short WH, et al. The change in ulnar variance with grip. J Hand Surg Am 1993;18(4):713–6.

5. Tomaino MM. The importance of the pronated grip x-ray view in evaluating ulnar variance. J Hand Surg Am 2000;25(2):352–7.

6. Tomaino MM, Rubin DA. The value of the pronated-grip view radiograph in assessing dynamic ulnar positive variance: a case report. Am J Orthop (Belle Mead NJ) 1999;28(3):180–1.

7. af Ekenstam FW, Palmer AK, Glisson RR. The load on the radius and ulna in different positions of the wrist and forearm. A cadaver study. Acta Orthop Scand 1984;55(3):363–5.

8. Pfaeffle HJ, Manson T, Fischer KJ. Axial loading alters ulnar variance and distal ulna load with forearm pronation. Pittsburgh Orthop J 1999;10:101–2.

9. Markolf KL, Tejwani SG, Benhaim P. Effects of wafer resection and hemiresection from the distal ulna on load-sharing at the wrist: a cadaveric study. J Hand Surg Am 2005;30(2):351–8.

10. Wnorowski DC, Palmer AK, Werner FW, et al. Anatomic and biomechanical analysis of the arthroscopic wafer procedure. Arthroscopy 1992;8(2): 204–12.

11. Feldon P, Terrono AL, Belsky MR. Wafer distal ulna resection for triangular fibrocartilage tears and/or ulna impaction syndrome. J Hand Surg Am 1992; 17(4):731–7.

12. Feldon P, Terrono AL, Belsky MR. The "wafer" procedure. Partial distal ulnar resection. Clin Orthop Relat Res 1992;275:124–9.

13. Baek GH, Chung MS, Lee YH, et al. Ulnar shortening osteotomy in idiopathic ulnar impaction syndrome. J Bone Joint Surg Am 2005;87(12):2649–54.

14. Chen WS, Shih CH. Ulnar variance and Kienbock's disease. An investigation in Taiwan. Clin Orthop Relat Res 1990;255:124–7.

15. Jung JM, Baek GH, Kim JH, et al. Changes in ulnar variance in relation to forearm rotation and grip. J Bone Joint Surg Br 2001;83(7):1029–33.

16. Kristensen SS, Thomassen E, Christensen F. Ulnar variance determination. J Hand Surg Br 1986; 11(2):255–7.

17. Kristensen SS, Thomassen E, Christensen F. Ulnar variance in Kienbock's disease. J Hand Surg Br 1986;11(2):258–60.

18. Nakamura R, Tanaka Y, Imaeda T, et al. The influence of age and sex on ulnar variance. J Hand Surg Br 1991;16(1):84–8.

19. Schuind FA, Linscheid RL, An KN, et al. A normal database of posteroanterior roentgenographic measurements of the wrist. J Bone Joint Surg Am 1992;74(9):1418–29.

20. Nakamura R, Horii E, Imaeda T, et al. The ulnocarpal stress test in the diagnosis of ulnar-sided wrist pain. J Hand Surg Br 1997;22(6):719–23.

21. Sachar K. Ulnar-sided wrist pain: evaluation and treatment of triangular fibrocartilage complex tears, ulnocarpal impaction syndrome, and lunotriquetral ligament tears. J Hand Surg Am 2008;33(9):1669–79.

22. Cerezal L, del Pinal F, Abascal F, et al. Imaging findings in ulnar-sided wrist impaction syndromes. Radiographics 2002;22(1):105–21.

23. Steinborn M, Schurmann M, Staebler A, et al. MR imaging of ulnocarpal impaction after fracture of the distal radius. AJR Am J Roentgenol 2003;181(1):195–8.

24. Imaeda T, Nakamura R, Shionoya K, et al. Ulnar impaction syndrome: MR imaging findings. Radiology 1996;201(2):495–500.

25. Palmer AK. Triangular fibrocartilage complex lesions: a classification. J Hand Surg Am 1989; 14(4):594–606.

26. Tomaino MM, Elfar J. Ulnar impaction syndrome. Hand Clin 2005;21(4):567–75.

27. Milch H. Cuff resection of the ulna for malunited Colles' fracture. J Bone Joint Surg 1941;23:311–3.

28. Barry JA, Macksoud WS. Cartilage-retaining wafer resection osteotomy of the distal ulna. Clin Orthop Relat Res 2008;466(2):396–401.

29. Pechlaner S. Dekompressionsosteotomie des ellenkopfes bei impingementbeschwerden im ulnaren handgelenkkompartiment. Operat Orthop Traumatol 1995;7:164–74 [in German].

30. Slade JF 3rd, Gillon TJ. Osteochondral shortening osteotomy for the treatment of ulnar impaction syndrome: a new technique. Tech Hand Up Extrem Surg 2007;11(1):74–82.

31. Berger RA, Cooney WP 3rd. Use of an ulnar head endoprosthesis for treatment of an unstable distal ulnar resection: review of mechanics, indications, and surgical technique. Hand Clin 2005;21(4):603–20, vii.

32. Bowers WH. Distal radioulnar joint arthroplasty: the hemiresection-interposition technique. J Hand Surg Am 1985;10(2):169–78.

33. Darrach W. Partial excision of the lower shaft of the ulna for deformity following Colles' fracture. Ann Surg 1913;57:764–5.

34. Watson HK, Ryu JY, Burgess RC. Matched distal ulnar resection. J Hand Surg Am 1986;11(6):812–7.

35. Tomaino MM, Gainer M, Towers JD. Carpal impaction with the ulnar styloid process: treatment with partial styloid resection. J Hand Surg Br 2001; 26(3):252–5.

36. Baek GH, Chung MS, Lee YH, et al. Ulnar shortening osteotomy in idiopathic ulnar impaction syndrome. Surgical technique. J Bone Joint Surg Am 2006; 88(Suppl 1 Pt 2):212–20.

37. Nishiwaki M, Nakamura T, Nagura T, et al. Ulnar-shortening effect on distal radioulnar joint pressure: a biomechanical study. J Hand Surg Am 2008;33(2):198–205.

38. Fricker R, Pfeiffer KM, Troeger H. Ulnar shortening osteotomy in posttraumatic ulnar impaction syndrome. Arch Orthop Trauma Surg 1996; 115(3–4):158–61.

39. Iwasaki N, Ishikawa J, Kato H, et al. Factors affecting results of ulnar shortening for ulnar impaction syndrome. Clin Orthop Relat Res 2007;465:215–9.

40. Lauder AJ, Luria S, Trumble TE. Oblique ulnar shortening osteotomy with a new plate and compression system. Tech Hand Up Extrem Surg 2007;11(1):66–73.

41. Moermans A, Degreef I, De Smet L. Ulnar shortening osteotomy for ulnar ideopathic impaction syndrome. Scand J Plast Reconstr Surg Hand Surg 2007;41(6): 310–4.

42. Chen F, Osterman AL, Mahony K. Smoking and bony union after ulna-shortening osteotomy. Am J Orthop (Belle Mead NJ) 2001;30(6):486–9.

43. Rayhack JM, Gasser SI, Latta LL, et al. Precision oblique osteotomy for shortening of the ulna. J Hand Surg Am 1993;18(5):908–18.

44. Constantine KJ, Tomaino MM, Herndon JH, et al. Comparison of ulnar shortening osteotomy and the wafer resection procedure as treatment for ulnar impaction syndrome. J Hand Surg Am 2000;25(1):55–60.

45. Bernstein MA, Nagle DJ, Martinez A, et al. A comparison of combined arthroscopic triangular fibrocartilage complex debridement and arthroscopic wafer distal ulna resection versus arthroscopic triangular fibrocartilage complex debridement and ulnar shortening osteotomy for ulnocarpal abutment syndrome. Arthroscopy 2004; 20(4):392–401.

The Sauvé-Kapandji Procedure: Indications and Tips for Surgical Success

Alberto Lluch, MD, PhD

KEYWORDS
- Wrist • Distal radioulnar joint • Arthrodesis
- Triangular fibrocartilage • Ulnocarpal impaction

Many procedures have been described for the management of the altered distal radioulnar joint (DRUJ), not only because there is no single procedure superior to another, but mainly because of a broad spectrum of pathology requiring different surgical techniques for each lesion.[1–3] The most common alterations of the DRUJ are joint incongruencies secondary to deformities of the distal radius from malunited fractures, distal radial epiphysiodesis, or Madelung deformities. Isolated joint instabilities after ruptures of the distal radioulnar ligaments are also common. Primary degenerative arthritis is unusual, although secondary arthritis may be observed after fractures of the distal radius or ulna involving the DRUJ. In other cases, the problems may be related to the "ulnocarpal joint" rather than the DRUJ, as in triangular fibrocartilage complex (TFCC) tears or the so-called "ulnocarpal impaction syndrome" when the ulna is longer than the radius.

Resection of the ulnar head was first described by Joseph François Malgaine in 1855,[4] and later popularized by William Darrach in 1912 and 1913.[5,6] It is an easy procedure to perform with early good functional results, although not free of complications if an excessive amount of ulna is excised.[7,8] These consist mainly of instability of the proximal ulna, loss of grip strength, and possible ulnar translation of the carpus in rheumatoid patients from loss of ulnar support. To avoid these possible complications, Bowers,[9] Watson and colleagues,[10] and Feldon and colleagues[11] described techniques of partial resection of the ulnar head while preserving the ulnar styloid and the ligaments inserting at its base.

In 1921, Baldwin[12] reported restoration of pronation and supination of the forearm after malunited distal radial fractures, after excision of a 2-cm segment of the ulna proximal to the DRUJ, thus creating a pseudoarthrosis.

In 1936, Louis Sauvé de Gonzagues and Mehmed Ibrahim Kapandji[13] described a similar technique, with the variant that a DRUJ arthrodesis was added to the pseudoarthrosis of the ulna. This technique was attributed to Lauenstein by Arthur Steindler[14] and for many years he was referred to as the author of the technique in the English medical literature.[15] What Lauenstein had actually described was a resection of the head of the ulna.[16]

The so-called Sauvé-Kapandji (S-K) technique had already been published, however, by Berry[17,18] in 1931. This procedure had been done the year before, the only difference being that instead of screws or Kirschner wires, a bone peg was used to stabilize the DRUJ arthrodesis.

Arthrodesis of the DRUJ has the advantage over complete ulnar head resection of preserving ulnar support of the wrist, because the distal radioulnar and ulnocarpal ligaments are preserved. It also allows for unlimited shortening of the ulnar head, which cannot always be done with resection

Adapted from Slutsky DJ. The Sauvé-Kapandji procedure. In: Lluch A, Garcia-Elias MD, editors. Principles and Practice of Wrist Surgery. Saunders-Elsevier, 2009. p. 335–44.
Institut Kaplan for Surgery of the Hand and Upper Extremity, Paseo Bonanova 9, 08022 Barcelona, Spain
E-mail address: albertolluch@institut-kaplan.com

Hand Clin 26 (2010) 559–572
doi:10.1016/j.hcl.2010.07.002
0749-0712/10/$ — see front matter © 2010 Elsevier Inc. All rights reserved.

arthroplasties that preserve the length of the styloid process of the ulna, such as the techniques described by Bowers,[9] Watson and colleagues,[10] and Feldon and colleagues.[11] Another advantage of the S-K technique is that the postoperative immobilization is shorter, which is an added benefit for the patient.

INDICATIONS

The S-K technique is indicated for the treatment of any pathology of the DRUJ and the so-called "ulnocarpal joint." It is most commonly indicated after malunited fractures of the distal end of the radius. If the radius fracture heals with some deformity, either dorsal or volar angulation, the DRUJ is not congruent and the patient complains of pain and limited forearm rotation. The same occur if the fracture of the distal radius heals with bone shortening, in which case the long ulna causes ulnocarpal impaction. Other times, the DRUJ is destroyed from a fracture of the sigmoid notch of the radius and less frequently from a fracture of the head of the ulna. The S-K technique allows for shortening of the ulna for treating ulnocarpal impaction, and recovery of forearm rotation. Severe distal radial angulations may need to be corrected to prevent adaptative carpal collapse deformities. Correcting the radial deformity is usually a priority, although both procedures can be performed at the same time, with the only drawback that this adds a technical difficulty to the procedure. In some very distal radial osteotomies, one is not able to stabilize the ulnar head to the radius with a screw, and may have to use Kirschner wires instead, which does not provide as solid stability.

The S-K technique is also indicated for the treatment of isolated DRUJ instabilities secondary to ligament ruptures. Ligament repair techniques do not always offer adequate joint stability[19] and require long periods of immobilization of the wrist and elbow, which may be very uncomfortable and disabling for the patient, and lead to a loss of forearm rotation in some cases.[20,21]

Chronic or difficult to repair TFCC tears can also be treated with a S-K procedure.[22] The patient can resume normal daily activities after the skin sutures are removed, because the screw provides for stabilization of the DRUJ, avoiding the long periods of immobilization needed after TFCC repairs. When the DRUJ is arthrodesed there are no strains into the TFCC, and lesions "spontaneously" repair if their vascularity allows. The author started treating chronic TFCC tears with the S-K technique after observing spontaneous healing of delayed unions of styloid fractures of the ulna after DRUJ arthrodesis (**Fig. 1**).

This technique can also be used for the treatment of early synovitis of the DRUJ in rheumatoid patients.[23-26] As a result from the arthrodesis, the synovitis permanently disappears, preventing rupture of the distal radioulnar and ulnocarpal ligaments. When the ulnar head is completely dislocated, the procedure does not provide ligamentous stability, because they have already been destroyed. The S-K procedure may be of benefit if a simultaneous radiolunate arthrodesis has to be performed in those cases of important ulnar translocation of the carpus, because more bone contact is obtained between the lunate and the distal radius and ulna. When the head of the ulna is completely dislocated, the only advantage of the S-K over the Darrach technique is that it achieves a better aesthetic result. It is preferred for women with thin wrists in which cases the normal prominence of the ulnar head, when the forearm is in pronation, is lost after ulnar head resection. This is more noticeable in wrists with some ulnar translocation of the carpus.

SURGICAL TECHNIQUE

An axillary block anesthesia is recommended, because it is better tolerated by the patient, and surgery may be done on an ambulatory basis. The surgical approach is done through a "V" incision with the vertex centered over the dorsal rim of the sigmoid notch of the radius, and with its distal and proximal arms directed anteriorly forming a 90-degree angle. The dorsal sensory branch of the ulnar nerve runs obliquely from proximal-volar to distal-dorsal at the level of the triquetrum, which can be identified and protected at the distal part of the incision. The fifth extensor compartment is divided longitudinally and the extensor digiti minimi tendon is retracted toward the radial side. By doing so, one has a better visualization of the dorsal edge of the sigmoid notch of the radius, and this prevents inadvertent injury to this small caliber tendon. The dorsal DRUJ capsule is divided longitudinally close to its insertion into the radius, and then peeled off for a few millimeters to allow for adequate exposure of sigmoid notch of the radius (**Fig. 2**). The extensor carpi ulnaris (ECU) tendon glides inside an osteofibrous tunnel just radial to the styloid process of the ulna, and is independent from the extensor retinaculum.[26] The ECU sheath should not be opened because it is an important DRUJ stabilizer.[27]

With the forearm in pronation, the joint cartilage and subchondral bone of the ulnar head facing the surgeon are removed, leaving a slightly convex surface of cancellous bone. This corresponds to that part of the ulnar head dorsal to the ECU

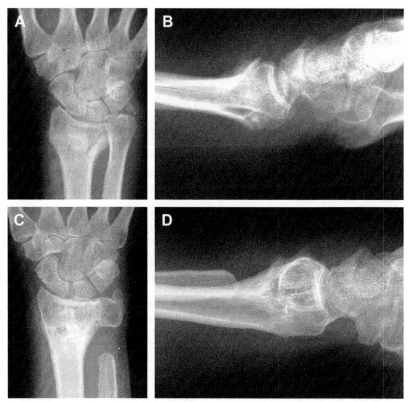

Fig. 1. (*A*) Posteroanterior radiograph of the wrist in a patient suffering from a painful DRUJ instability and pseudoarthrosis of the styloid process of the ulna after having sustained a Colles fracture. (*B*) Lateral radiograph of the same wrist demonstrating a 39-degree dorsal angulation of the distal joint surface of the radius. (*C*) Posteroanterior radiograph showing that the pseudoarthrosis of the ulnar styloid healed spontaneously after the DRUJ arthrodesis. A slightly larger than average segment of ulna was removed, because it had to be used as a bone graft. The cylinder of ulna bone that was excised was later split in half, and both pieces placed side by side as a buttress, in the space of the dorsal open wedge radius osteotomy. (*D*) Lateral radiograph showing DRUJ arthrodesis, almost full correction of the distal radius, and good alignment of the ulna at the level pseudoarthrosis.

tendon sheath (**Fig. 3**). The ulnar head is perforated with a 3.2-mm drill, with the entrance at the center of the denuded ulnar head and the exit anterior to the ECU sheath (**Fig. 4**). The direction of the drill should be perpendicular to the long axis of the radius and ulna. The triangular skin flap should be retracted to visualize and confirm that the exit of the drill bit is just anterior the sixth compartment of the extensor retinaculum. With a small knife blade, the puncture wound into the extensor retinaculum produced by the drill bit should be enlarged longitudinally, to later facilitate easy identification of the screw entrance point.

Next, the head of the ulna is osteotomized just proximal to where the joint cartilage ends. The osteotomized head of the ulna can then be displaced and rotated into supination, allowing visualization of the sigmoid notch of the radius and the proximal ulnar stump (**Fig. 5**). The osteotomy can be done

with an oscillating saw using a thin blade with fine teeth to prevent excessive seeding of bone particles into the soft tissues. However, I prefer to use small bone rongeur because there is no cortical bone in this area, and the osteotomy can be easily done by circumferentially nibbling the ulna from the starting point.

Next, a segment of the proximal ulnar stump should be removed. In those cases in which there is no length discrepancy between radius and ulna, only 5 mm of ulna should be removed. If the ulna is longer than the radius an additional segment of the ulna, equivalent to the length discrepancy, should be removed. In young patients in whom more than 5 mm of ulna has to be removed for treating a positive ulnar variance, the dorsal cortex of the proximal ulna can be quite sharp if a power tool has been used for the osteotomy and it should be rounded off to prevent impingement against the

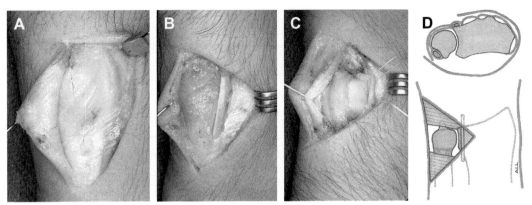

Fig. 2. (A) A "V" incision over the ulnar head is done. After hinging the flap toward the ulnar side, the extensor retinaculum can easily be visualized. (B) The fifth extensor retinaculum is longitudinally divided to expose the extensor digiti minimi tendon, which is later retracted toward the radial side. (C) The dorsal radioulnar joint capsule is longitudinally divided next to its insertion into the dorsal rim of the sigmoid notch of the radius. Joint synovectomy should be done when required, as in this case. (D) The top drawing shows the cross-section anatomy of the DRUJ. The forearm is in pronation, and the ulnar head is covered by the DRUJ capsule and the extensor retinaculum. The fifth extensor compartment stabilizes the extensor digiti minimi tendon at the most ulnar border of the distal radius. Extensor carpi ulnaris tendon is stabilized by its own sheath, separate from the extensor retinaculum, lateral to the styloid process of the ulna. In the bottom drawing, one can see the ulnar head after the extensor retinaculum has been ulnarly reflected and the dorsal radioulnar capsule removed. Division of the fifth extensor compartment allows a radial displacement of the extensor digiti minimi tendon, with improved exposure of the sigmoid notch of the radius.

radius or even rupture of a finger extensor tendon from friction against a sharp bony edge[28] during the early postoperative period. In time, the proximal ulna stump rounds off and also suffers some bone reabsortion. Bone excision of the proximal ulna should be done without damaging the insertions of the pronator quadrates (PQ), flexor carpi ulnaris (FCU), and ECU muscles, interosseous

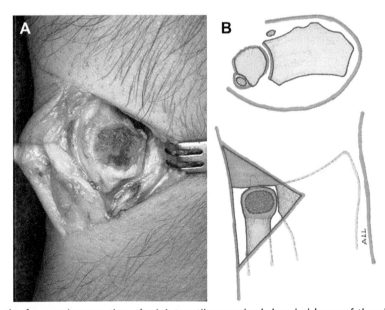

Fig. 3. (A) With the forearm in pronation, the joint cartilage and subchondral bone of the ulnar head facing the surgeon are removed, leaving a slightly convex surface of cancellous bone. (B) Schematic drawings showing the cartilage removal in cross-section and viewed from the top. (*Adapted from* Lluch A, Garcia-Elias MD. The Sauvé-Kapandji procedure. In: Slutsky DJ, editor. Principles and practice of wrist surgery. Philadelphia: Saunders-Elsevier; 2009. p. 335–44; with permission.)

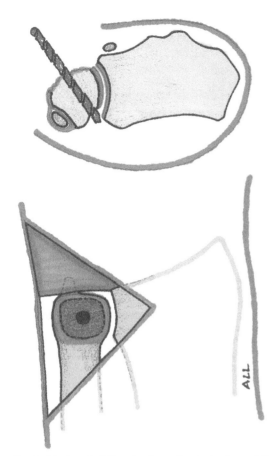

Fig. 4. The head of the ulna is perforated using a 3.2-mm drill bit, with the entrance at the center of the denuded ulnar head, exiting laterally to the styloid process and ECU sheath. The direction of the drill should be perpendicular to the long axis of the radius and ulna. (*Adapted from* Lluch A, Garcia-Elias MD. The Sauvé-Kapandji procedure. In: Slutsky DJ, editor. Principles and practice of wrist surgery. Philadelphia: Saunders-Elsevier; 2009. p. 335–44; with permission.)

membrane, and ECU tendon sheath into the proximal ulna. Retractors should be small and placed very carefully around the proximal ulna, and all resection should be done through the space created after the ulnar head has been displaced anteriorly, while rotating the radius into pronation and supination. After this is done, one should remove all bone debris and the periosteum of the segment of ulna that has already been removed.

The joint cartilage and subchondral bone of the sigmoid notch of the radius are then excised. Because the joint surface is slightly concave, it is difficult to bite into it with a bone rongeur. The procedure is facilitated if one starts at the angle formed by the union of the dorsal cortex and the dorsal rim of the sigmoid notch. Removal of the cartilage and subchondral bone can later be continued with a bone rongeur and a curette.

A malleolar lag screw is inserted into the head of the ulna, in a reverse direction, through the previously made drill hole. The entrance of the screw should be just anterior to the compartment for the ECU tendon, and introduced until its tip protrudes a few millimeters from the center of the denuded surface of the head of the ulna (**Fig. 6**). Using the screwdriver, the head of the ulna is reduced opposite to the radius until the protruding tip of the screw is placed at the center of the sigmoid notch of the radius. Before inserting the screw into the radius, one should carefully check the correct position of the head of the ulna in relation to the radius. The most distal part of the ulnar head should be about 2 mm shorter than ulnar edge of the radius. A slightly shorter ulnar head prevents ulnocarpal impingement and damage to the triangular fibrocartilage, and places the ulnocarpal ligaments under slight tension. The distal radial joint surface may be difficult to visualize, because its ulnar edge is covered by the radial insertion of the triangular fibrocartilage. Because it is very important not to arthrodese the ulna head in a position longer than the radius, one may need partially to detach the dorsal radioulnar ligament for more precise identification of the distal radial joint. The self-tapping malleolar screw is introduced through the distal end of the radius, perpendicular to the long axis of the bone, without the need of drilling. The screw should be from 35 to 40 mm in length, depending on the size of the wrist. In case of doubt, the radius should be drilled first and the length of the screw to be inserted measured with a depth gauge. It should not protrude through the radial cortex because this may cause injury from friction to the abductor pollicis longus tendon. The screw is advanced into the radius until the bone surfaces to be arthrodesed have been moderately compressed and the head of the screw is slightly introduced into the head of the ulna (**Fig. 7**). During the final turns of the screwdriver, the head of the ulna should be stabilized to prevent rotation when countersinking the head of the screw into the bone. After the radius and ulna have been fixed, one should check for a possible malrotation of the head of the ulna and the bone space created. The head of the ulna is not rotated when the osteotomized surfaces of the ulna are parallel to each other. The forearm is rotated to confirm that full pronation and supination can be obtained without impingement of the osteotomized ends of the

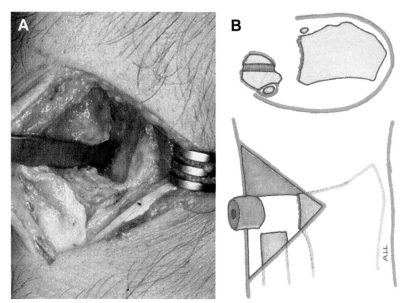

Fig. 5. (*A, B*) The head of the ulna is osteotomized at the level of the neck, and later displaced and rotated into supination allowing visualization of the sigmoid notch of the radius. A segment of the proximal ulna is excised and the joint cartilage and subchondral bone of the sigmoid notch of the radius are removed. (*Adapted from* Lluch A, Garcia-Elias MD. The Sauvé-Kapandji procedure. In: Slutsky DJ, editor. Principles and practice of wrist surgery. Philadelphia: Saunders-Elsevier; 2009. p. 335–44; with permission.)

ulna. The bone gap should not exceed 5 mm. Take into consideration that one is exploring the gap with the forearm in pronation, which is slightly larger when the forearm is supinated.

Fluoroscopic examination can be used to determine the position of the head of the ulna in relation to the radius and the position and length of the screw. In recent years I have also used double

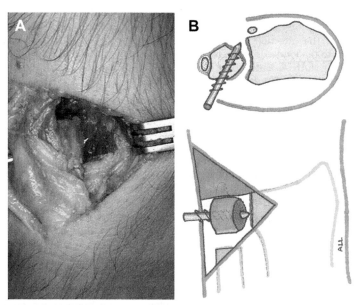

Fig. 6. (*A, B*) A malleolar screw is inserted perpendicular to the head of the ulna through the previously made drill hole, although in the opposite direction: the entrance of the screw corresponds to the exit of the drill. The entrance of the screw should be just anterior to the compartment of the ECU tendon, and introduced until its tip protrudes about 3 mm from the center of the denuded surface of the head of the ulna. (*Adapted from* Lluch A, Garcia-Elias MD. The Sauvé-Kapandji procedure. In: Slutsky DJ, editor. Principles and practice of wrist surgery. Philadelphia: Saunders-Elsevier; 2009. p. 335–44; with permission.)

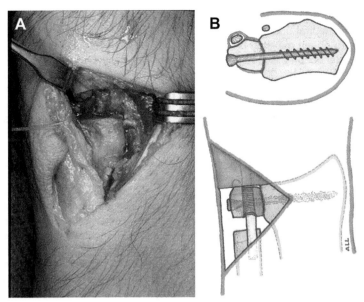

Fig. 7. (*A, B*) The screw is advanced until the bone surfaces to be arthrodesed have been compressed and the head of the screw is slightly introduced into the head of the ulna. The bone gap of the osteotomized ulna should measure about 5 mm, and the ECU tendon remain at the dorsum. (*Adapted from* Lluch A, Garcia-Elias MD. The Sauvé-Kapandji procedure. In: Slutsky DJ, editor. Principles and practice of wrist surgery. Philadelphia: Saunders-Elsevier; 2009. p. 335–44; with permission.)

thread compression screws, which have the advantage that they can be introduced around a temporary Kirschner wire and their head is left buried inside the bone. However, I am still in favor of using malleolar lag screws because they can be inserted into the radius without previous bone drilling and provide the highest compression and best stability.

The dorsal capsule and the dorsal radioulnar ligament do not need to be sutured because the distal radioulnar arthrodeses makes this unnecessary. The extensor digity minimy tendon is replaced into the fifth extensor compartment and the extensor retinaculum and the distal antebrachial fascia are sutured with interrupted sutures, using reabsorbable colorless material, such as polydioxanone (1 metric; 5–0 United States Pharmacopeia [USP]). The skin is closed with monofilament sutures, such as polypropylene or polyamide (0.7 metric; 6–0 USP). The wound edges should be loosely closed to avoid excessive skin pressure, and to allow for any postoperative bleeding to be absorbed by the gauze, rather than forming a subcutaneous hematoma. Steri-strips can be placed over the skin edges to prevent the gauze from adhering to the wound.

The hand and forearm are covered with a thin layer of cast padding, and a plaster bandage is loosely applied. Plaster is the only type of bandage that adapts to the flat shape of the hand and wrist,

without the risk of applying excessive global pressure, as may occur with a bulky compressive dressing. Pressure is applied by the surgeon's hand only over the surgical area on the dorsum and ulnar side of the wrist. After the plaster has hardened, the tourniquet is both released and removed at once, while the hand is maintained in maximum elevation. The hand should be maintained elevated over the axillary level at all times, particularly after the release of the tourniquet. If the skin is loosely closed, a plaster bandage applied, and the hand is elevated, there is no need to place drains or fear of hematoma formation.

POSTOPERATIVE CARE

The wrist is immobilized with a circular plaster bandage for 7 to 10 days. The patient is allowed to perform supination and pronation of the forearm inside the plaster cast, but this may be somewhat limited because of pain and plaster bandage constraints. After the bandage and the skin sutures are removed, the wrist is left free, and the patient is instructed to bring the forearm into maximal pronation and supination. The patient should not be continuously rotating the forearm, because this causes unnecessary inflammation and pain at the site of the pseudoarthrosis. He or she should rotate the forearm until maximal supination is achieved, and maintain it in this position for a while. After resting it temporarily in neutral position, the opposite should be done to obtain maximal pronation. Forearm rotation is better accomplished by passive mobilization with the elbow flexed 90 degrees. It is very important to avoid excessive inflammation at the pseudoarthrosis because this leads to pain, impaired mobility, increased collagenoblastic activity, and longer recovery time, and increases the chances of ossification or fibrous union at the pseudoarthrosis. If this occurs, the patient may benefit from a few days of rest and the intake of anti-inflammatory medication, preferably steroids, such as dexametasone, 1 mg three times a day for 3 days, followed by 1 mg each morning for an additional 3 to 4 days. The period of rest and steroid intake can be repeated if inflammation reoccurs. Within a postoperative period of approximately 3 weeks the patient achieves full pronation and supination of the forearm with minimal discomfort. However, during the first few weeks he or she may experience pain when carrying objects with the elbow flexed and the forearm in neutral position, because the weight of the object displaces the radius against the flexed ulna. Pain, with a feeling of bone snapping, can also be experienced when rotating the forearm from slight pronation to supination, and vice versa, from impingement of the stump of the osteotomized ulna against the ulnar border of the radius, particularly when carrying heavy objects.

RESULTS

Seventy patients who underwent the previously described technique were reviewed on an average of 8 years after surgery (from 3–12.5 years). Thirty-eight were women and 32 were men; one woman who presented with a Madelung deformity underwent surgery in both wrists. The average patient's age was 40 years, ranging from 25 to 70 years of age. The indications for surgery were DRUJ instability or incongruency after fractures of the distal radius in 44 wrists, primary DRUJ osteoarthritis in 3 wrists, isolated DRUJ instabilities secondary to ligament injuries in 10 wrists, rupture of the TFCC in 3 wrists, rheumatoid arthritis in 10 wrists, and Madelung deformity in 3 wrists. A simultaneous corrective osteotomy of the distal radius was performed in 10 wrists: 8 of the 23 wrists were sequelae after a fracture of the distal radius and 2 wrists with a Madelung deformity. Radioulnar arthrodesis was obtained in all cases, because optimal stability and bone contact were provided by the compression lag screw.

Radiocarpal joint mobility was not altered by the procedure, and all patients regained full wrist joint mobility shortly after the procedure. Only the 10 patients in whom a corrective osteotomy of the distal radius was performed required a longer postoperative period to recover full joint mobility, mainly wrist flexion, because of postoperative fibrosis of dorsal capsular structures. However, the arch of extension and flexion was moved to a more flexed position, because the dorsal inclination of the distal radial joint was corrected by the osteotomy.

Full pronation and supination was regained in all patients, except for two who had minimal restriction of supination. Calcification at the osteotomy site was observed in four cases, three of whom had a simultaneous distal radial osteotomy performed. Only two out of the four patients required excision of the calcification, because this caused restriction of forearm rotation. Three other patients complained of pain and presented inflammatory signs at the site of the pseudoarthrosis with intensity and duration longer than the average, which generally speaking was for about 3 weeks. Symptoms disappeared on an average of 3 months, after having been treated with short periods of rest and anti-inflammatory steroids.

When explored with the forearm in neutral position and the elbow flexed, all patients had increased passive displaceability of the proximal ulnar stump, although it was painless. However, when holding objects or asked actively to stabilize the wrist, the proximal ulna became stable from contraction of the PQ, FCU, and ECU muscles. At the time of exploration, on an average of 6.5 years after the procedure, none of the patients complained of painful instability throughout the entire range of pronosupination while holding heavy objects with their hands. All patients returned to their previous occupations.

POSSIBLE COMPLICATIONS

Just as with any surgical procedure there can be complications, but only three are directly related to the S-K procedure: (1) nonunion or delayed union of the arthrodesis, (2) fibrous or osseous union at the pseudoarthrosis, and (3) painful instability of the proximal ulna stump. The first two are not of much concern because they can be easily addressed. However, a painful instability of the proximal ulna stump can cause a serious disability, which in most cases can be very difficult to correct. Such complications can be prevented if one follows a careful surgical technique.[22,29,30]

Nonunion or Delayed Union of the Distal Radioulnar Arthrodesis

This does not occur if a malleolar or other compression lag screw is used for internal fixation, because it provides excellent stability and compression of the bone surfaces. Some authors recommend using a segment of the ulna that has been resected as a bone graft.[31–34] I do not recommend interposing a bone graft between the radius and ulna, because this creates an unnecessary barrier of devascularized tissue, particularly if cortical bone is used. There are no strains or transmission forces through the head of the ulna and therefore it is very rare to observe a pseudoarthrosis. Rothwell and colleagues[35] have even proposed to stabilize the DRUJ with a screw without formal removal of the joint cartilage and without postoperative immobilization. Six of their 22 operated patients presented with an asymptomatic nonunion. The above report proves that hardly any forces are transmitted through the DRUJ after the ulna has been proximally osteotomized. Therefore, 3 to 4 weeks postoperative immobilization, as recommended by many authors, is unnecessary, aside for adding discomfort to the patient.

Following Kapandji's recommendation,[36,37] most surgeons favor the use of two screws, or one screw and a Kirschner wire, for the internal fixation. It is true that the head of the ulna can rotate around the axis of the screw during insertion, which should be controlled by the surgeon, but this never occurs after the joint surfaces are engaged under compression. The youngest patient in our series, a 25-year-old professional motorcycle racer with a TFCC tear and painful instability of the DRUJ, participated in a competition 3 weeks after the procedure without any complications.

Proubasta and colleagues[38] proposed the use of a Herbert screw to avoid prominence of the head of the screw, but there is the risk of not providing enough compression when used in osteoporotic or partially destroyed bones, such as those affected with rheumatoid arthritis.

Fibrous or Osseous Union at the Pseudoarthrosis

The use of power tools facilitates the osteotomy of the ulna, mainly in young male patients with hard cortical bone, although the disadvantage may be seeding of the wound with bone debris. It is recommended to use a bone rongeur to perform both the osteotomy and the excision of a segment of ulna at the level of the neck of the ulna, where the cortical bone is very thin. In all cases, all bone debris and the periosteum of the ulna at the level of the pseudoarthrosis should be removed. However, Carter and Stuart[39] found no differences in the two groups of patients in which the periosteum had or had not been removed.

This complication should not be a major concern, because it can be resolved by a second operation, using a limited approach with minimal tissue trauma to remove the fibrous tissue or the calcification with a bone rongeur. The patients who underwent simultaneous corrective osteotomy of the distal radial metaphysis and a S-K procedure had more difficulties to regain rotation of the forearm, probably from increased discomfort related to the surgical trauma.

Following the initial description of the technique, some surgeons remove larger amounts of ulna,

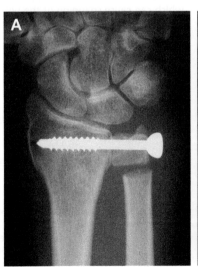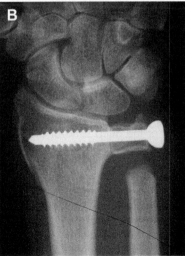

Fig. 8. (A) The pseudoarthrosis should be created just proximal to the ulnar head cartilage, leaving a bone defect no larger than 5 mm. (B) With time, the proximal ulna stump rounds off and slightly reabsorbs, creating a larger bone defect.

and interposing a flap of the PQ muscle, with the aim of decreasing the probability of fibrous union at the pseudoarthrosis.[36,38–41] However, it is known from clinical experience, after treating fractures of the scaphoid, humerus, ulna, tibia, and so forth, that a pseudoarthrosis occurs if mobility is maintained between the fractured bone ends, regardless of the size of the bone gap.

Painful Instability of the Proximal Ulna Stump

Most authors have reported good to excellent results after the S-K technique,[42–49] whereas some have been concerned with the creation of painful instability of the proximal ulnar stump. The pseudoarthrosis should be created just proximal to the ulnar head, leaving a bone defect no larger than 5 mm (**Fig. 8**). The reason for this is to make the pseudoarthrosis as close as possible to the axis of rotation of the forearm, which runs obliquely from the center of the radial head proximally to the center of the ulnar head distally (**Fig. 9**). An osteotomy at a more proximal level causes a divergence of movements between the proximal ulna and the head of the ulna, which has already been fixed to the radius. Another reason for creating a more distal pseudoarthrosis is so as not to disturb the static and dynamic structures, which provide stability to the proximal ulna: the PQ, ECU, and FCU muscles and interosseous membrane insertions (**Fig. 10**).[27,50–53] The deep head of the PQ is the main dynamic stabilizer of the proximal ulna[53] and should not be stripped from the ulna and used as interposition between both ends of the ulna (**Fig. 11**). Very proximal resections, and other others as large as 2.5 cm, have been recommended by some authors, with the main inconvenience of leaving the proximal ulnar stump without stabilizing structures. It has been observed that the degree of instability increases as more bone is resected.[54]

There is a relatively flat triangular-shaped surface proximal to the sigmoid articular facet of the radius for the ulna, measuring on average 20.5 ± 1.3 mm in length, which serves for insertion of the muscle fibers of the deep head of the PQ muscle.[26] Proximally to this flat surface area, the ulnar side of the radius becomes a ridge serving for insertion to the interosseous membrane. This triangular-shaped flat surface, just proximal to the sigmoid notch of the radius is, from a mechanical point of view, the best place to have the proximal stump of the ulna to have contact with the radius (**Fig. 12**). If the ulnar stump is more proximally located, the chances of creating a painful snapping around the ridge of the radius are increased. The reason why a painful instability of

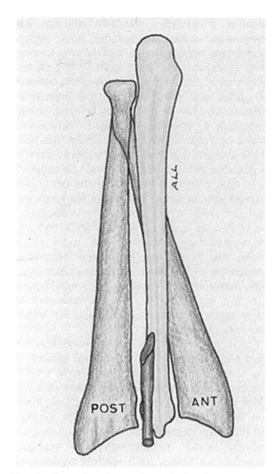

Fig. 9. The axis of rotation of the forearm runs obliquely, from the center of the radial head proximally to the center of the ulnar head distally. Creating a distal pseudoarthrosis minimizes lateral translation of the proximal ulna when pronating the forearm, which can cause snapping of the ulna over the radial crest when the osteotomy is done too proximally.

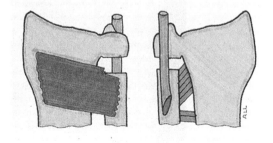

Fig. 10. The structures stabilizing the proximal ulna should not be damaged during the procedure: interosseus membrane, pronator quadrates, and flexor carpi ulnaris muscles anteriorly, and extensor carpi ulnaris muscle and sheath posteriorly. (*Adapted from* Lluch A, Garcia-Elias MD. The Sauvé-Kapandji procedure. In: Slutsky DJ, editor. Principles and practice of wrist surgery. Philadelphia: Saunders-Elsevier; 2009. p. 335–44; with permission.)

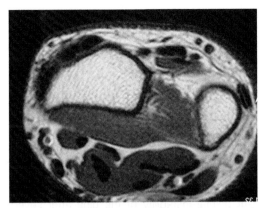

Fig. 11. Both heads of the pronator quadratus muscle, mainly the deep head, are the most important dynamic stabilizers of the proximal ulna stump.

the proximal ulna stump is seen more commonly observed after the S-K procedure as opposed to the Darrach is probably because the osteotomy of the ulna is done more proximally in the S-K procedure.

It is also very important to leave the ECU sheath undisturbed and dorsal to the pseudoarthrosis, for added stabilization.[26,27] The entrance of the screw should be anterior to the ECU sheath, allowing for the ECU to remain dorsal to the pseudoarthrosis further preventing dorsal instability of the proximal ulna. Because the surgery is usually done with the forearm in pronation, it is not uncommon inadvertently to place the entrance of the screw dorsal to the ECU, leaving the ECU in a lateral or even anterior position in relation to the pseudoarthrosis (**Fig. 13**).

The interosseous membrane is also a radioulnar stabilizer, preventing excessive translation of the radius in relation to the ulna during supination and pronation of the forearm, and should not be disturbed while resecting a segment of ulna (**Fig. 14**).

For the prevention or treatment of proximal ulna instability several additional procedures have been

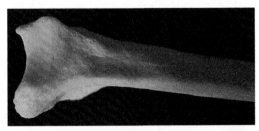

Fig. 12. Proximal to the sigmoid joint of the radius is a triangular-shaped flat surface, which from the mechanical point of view is the best place for the proximal stump of the ulna to have contact with the radius.

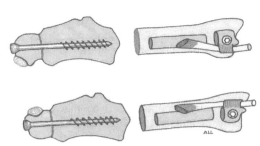

Fig. 13. Because the surgery is done with the forearm in pronation, it is not uncommon inadvertently to place the entrance of the screw dorsal to the ECU, as shown in the top drawing. The ulnar head should be arthrodesed in a position of supination to maintain the ECU tendon dorsally for added stability of the proximal ulna, as depicted in the bottom drawing. (*Adapted from* Lluch A, Garcia-Elias MD. The Sauvé-Kapandji procedure. In: Slutsky DJ, editor. Principles and practice of wrist surgery. Philadelphia: Saunders-Elsevier; 2009. p. 335–44; with permission.)

proposed, such as creating a loop around the ulna with a palmaris longus tendon graft[55] or tenodesing the proximal ulna stump with a slip of the FCU or ECU tendons.[56,57] The latter two, using tendon slips distally inserted into the carpus, have the theoretical disadvantage of limiting radial inclination of the carpus if they are excessively tight or being completely inefficient if the wrist is placed into ulnar inclination.

TENOTOMY OF THE BRACHIALIS MUSCLE INTO THE ULNA

Several authors have demonstrated that when the elbow is flexed and the hand is holding an object, the DRUJ is important in the transmission of

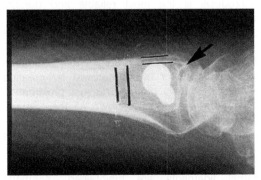

Fig. 14. Lateral radiograph demonstrating the best tips for a successful S-K procedure. The head of the ulna is fixed to the center of the sigmoid notch of the radius with a single melleolar lag screw. Bone resection should be less than 5 mm in length. The styloid process of the ulna and the ECU tendon should be located at the dorsum, as shown by an arrow.

loads[58–60] because both the radius and ulna are brought into flexion by the elbow flexor muscles. If the ulna has been osteotomized proximal to the joint, the proximal ulna stump impinges into the radius. The brachialis is the only muscle inserting into the ulna, and on contraction it causes radioulnar impingement. Based on this functional anatomy observation, it was hypothesized that sectioning the brachialis insertion into the ulna would prevent impingement of the ulna against the radius. Five patients presenting with a painful proximal ulna stump, after an S-K procedure performed elsewhere, have been referred to the author because the patients were not asymptomatic after a variety of soft tissue stabilization procedures. All five patients underwent two or three infiltrations of the brachialis muscle, during a 1-year period, with botulinic toxin to paralyze the muscle and ascertain the effectiveness of the procedure. Different functional tests and force measurements were done during that period of time, and all patients related a complete remission of the painful radioulnar impingement. At the end of the trial all patients decided to have the brachialis tendon insertion into the ulna surgically divided. After this was done, the patient held objects only with the radius, mainly from the contraction of the biceps and the brachioradialis muscles. The proximal ulna stump remained unstable, but did not impinge against the radius when holding or manipulating objects. Although some elbow flexion had to be lost after the muscle tenotomy, it was difficult to measure this in our group of patients, because the pain during the preoperative period limited full elbow flexion force.

SUMMARY

Arthrodesis is the most reliable and durable surgical procedure for the treatment of a joint disorder, with the main disadvantage of loss of motion of the fused joint. The DRUJ can be arthrodesed, whereas forearm pronation and supination are maintained or even improved by creating a pseudoarthrosis of the ulna just proximal to the arthrodesis. This is known as the "Sauvé-Kapandji" procedure.

The S-K differs from the Darrach procedure in that it preserves ulnar support of the wrist, because the distal radioulnar ligaments and ulnocarpal ligaments are maintained. Aesthetic appearance is also superior after the S-K procedure, because the normal prominence of the ulnar head, most noticeable when the forearm is in pronation, is not lost. However, the S-K is not void of possible complications, such as nonunion or delayed union of the arthrodesis, fibrous or osseous union at the pseudoarthrosis, and painful instability at the proximal ulna stump. All of these can be prevented if a careful surgical technique is used.

ACKNOWLEDGMENTS

The author thanks his partner Marc Garcia-Elias, MD, PhD, for allowing review of his patients treated with the Sauvé-Kapandji procedure. The author also thanks his nephew and partner Alex Lluch, MD, for performing sectioning of the brachialis muscle tendon into the ulna for the treatment painful instability of the ulna after several other treatments had previously failed.

REFERENCES

1. Minami A, Ogino T, Minami M. Treatment of distal radioulnar disorders. J Hand Surg Am 1987;12: 189–96.
2. Lichtman DM, Ganocy TK, Kim DC. The indications for and techniques and outcomes of ablative procedures of the distal ulna. The Darrach resection, hemiresection, matched resection, and Sauvé-Kapandji procedure. Hand Clin 1998;14(2):265–77.
3. Lluch A. Patología de la articulación radio-cubital distal. In: Herrera Rodríguez A, editor. Actualizaciones en cirugía ortopédica y traumatología. Barcelona (Spain): Mason; 2000. p. 185–97.
4. Malgaine JF. Traité des fractures et des luxations, vol. 2. Paris: JB Brailliére; 1855.
5. Darrach W. Anterior dislocation of the head of the ulna. Ann Surg 1912;56:802–3.
6. Darrach W. Partial excision of lower shaft of the ulna for deformity following Colles's fracture. Ann Surg 1913;57:764–5.
7. Field J, Majkowski RJ, Leslie IJ. Poor results of Darrach's procedure after wrist injuries. J Bone Joint Surg Br 1993;75:53–7.
8. Garcia-Elias M. Failed ulnar head resection: prevention and treatment. J Hand Surg Br 2002;27:470–80.
9. Bowers WH. Distal radioulnar joint arthroplasty. The hemiresection interposition technique. J Hand Surg Am 1985;10:169–78.
10. Watson HK, Ryu J, Burgess R. Matched distal ulnar resection. J Hand Surg Am 1986;11:812–7.
11. Feldon P, Terrono AL, Belsky MR. Wafer distal ulna resection for triangular fibrocartilage tears and/or ulna impaction syndrome. J Hand Surg Am 1992; 17:731–7.
12. Baldwin WI. Orthopaedic surgery of the hand and wrist. In: Jones R, editor. Orthopaedic surgery of injuries. London: Henry Frowde and Hodder & Stoughton; 1921. p. 241–82.
13. Sauvé L, Kapandji M. Nouvelle technique de traitement chirurgical des luxations récidivantes isolées

de l'extrémité inférieure du cubitus. J Chirurgie 1936;47:589–94 [in French].

14. Steindler A. The traumatic deformities and disabilities of the upper extremity. Illinois (IL): Charles C. Thomas; 1946.

15. Buck-Gramcko D. On the priorities of publication of some operative procedures on the distal end of the ulna. J Hand Surg Br 1990;15:416–20.

16. Lauenstein C. Zur Behandlung der nach karpaler Vorderarmfraktur zurückbleibenden Störung der Pro-und Supinations-bewegung. Centralblatt für Chir 1887;23:433–5 [in German].

17. Berry JA. Chronic subluxation of the distal radio-ulnar articulation. Br J Surg 1931;18:526–7.

18. Arandes JM, Ferreres A. Letter to the editor. J Hand Surg Br 1999;24:755.

19. Petersen MS, Adams BD. Biomechanical evaluation of distal radioulnar reconstructions. J Hand Surg Am 1993;18:328–34.

20. Szabo RM. Distal radioulnar joint instability. J Bone Joint Surg Am 2006;88:884–94.

21. Garcia-Elias M. Radioulnar instability. Curr Orthop 1999;13:283–9.

22. Lluch A, Garcia-Elias M. Arthrodesis of the distal radio-ulnar joint with pseudoarthrosis of the distal ulna: the Sauvé-Kapandji procedure. Paris: Elsevier; 2004.

23. Alnot JY, Faroux L. Synovectomy realignment stabilization in the rheumatoid wrist. In: Simmen BR, Hagena F-W, editors. The wrist in rheumatoid arthritis. Rheumatology. Basel (Switzerland): Karger; 1992. p. 72–96.

24. Vincent KA, Szabo RM, Agee JM. The Sauve-Kapandji procedure for reconstruction of the rheumatoid distal radioulnar joint. J Hand Surg Am 1993;18:978–83.

25. Alnot JY, Faroux L. La synovectomie réaxation stabilisation du poignet rhumatoïde incluant l'opération de Sauvé Kapandji. In: Tubiana R, editor. Traité de chirurgie de la main, vol. 5. Paris: Masson; 1995. p. 442–52.

26. Obry C, Tran Van F, Fardellon P, et al. L'association synovectomie postérieure, réaxation carpienne et opération de Sauvé Kapandji dans le traitement du poignet rhumatoïde. A propos de 60 cas. La Main 1996;1:299–306 [in French].

27. Garcia-Elias M. Soft tissue anatomy and relationship about the distal ulna. Hand Clin 1998;14:165–76.

28. Spinner M, Kaplan EB. Extensor carpi ulnaris. Its relationship to the stability of the distal radio-ulnar joint. Clin Orthop 1970;68:124–9.

29. Wada T, Ogino T, Ishii S. Closed rupture of a finger extensor following the Sauve-Kapandji procedure: a case report. J Hand Surg Am 1997;22:705–7.

30. Lluch AL, Garcia-Elias M. The Sauvé-Kapandji procedure: technical considerations. Orthopeadic Surgical Techniques 1995;9:67–70.

31. Lluch AL, Garcia-Elias M. The Sauvé-Kapandji procedure. In: Slutsky DR, editor. Principles and practice of wrist surgery. Philadelphia: Elsevier; 2010. p. 335–44.

32. Kapandji IA. The Kapandji-Sauvé operation: its techniques and indications in non-rheumatoid arthritis. Ann Chir Main 1986;5(3):181–93.

33. Nakamura R, Tsunoda K, Watanabe K, et al. The Sauvé-Kapandji procedure for chronic dislocation of the distal radio-ulnar joint with destruction of the articular surface. J Hand Surg Br 1992;17:127–32.

34. Minami A, Suzuki K, Suenaga N, et al. The Sauvé-Kapandji procedure for osteoarthritis of the distal radioulnar joint. J Hand Surg Am 1995;20:602–8.

35. Rothwell AG, O'Neill L, Cragg K. Sauvé-Kapandji procedure for disorders of the distal radioulnar joint: a simplified technique. J Hand Surg Am 1996;21:771–7.

36. Kapandji AI. Technique and indications of the Kapandji-Sauvé procedure in non-rheumatoid diseases of the wrist. In: Nakamura R, Linscheid RL, Miura T, editors. Wrist disorders. Current concepts and challenges. Tokyo: Springer-Verlag; 1992. p. 275–84.

37. Kapandji AI. Amélioration technique de l'operation Kapandji-Sauvé, dite "Technique III". Ann Chir Main 1998;17:78–86 [in French].

38. Proubasta IR, De Frutos AG, Salo GB, et al. Sauvé-Kapandji procedure using the herbert canulated bone screw. Tech Hand Up Extrem Surg 2000;4(2):120–6.

39. Carter PB, Stuart PR. The Sauve-Kapandji procedure for post-traumatic disorders of the distal radio-ulnar joint. J Bone Joint Surg Br 2000;82:1013–8.

40. Slater RR. The Sauvé-Kapandji procedure. J Hand Surg Am 2008;33:1632–8.

41. Ruby LK, Ferenz CC, Dell PC. The pronator quadratus interposition transfer: an adjunct to resection arthroplasty of the distal radioulnar joint. J Hand Surg Am 1996;21:60–5.

42. Szabo RM. Sauve Kapandji procedure. In: Gelberman RH, editor. Master techniques in orthopaedic surgery. The wrist. Philadelphia: Lippincott Williams & Wilkins; 2010. p. 399–409.

43. Taleisnik J. The whist. New York: Churchill Livingstone; 1985.

44. Sanders RA, Frederick HA, Hontas RB. The Sauvé-Kapandji procedure: a salvage operation for the distal radioulnar joint. J Hand Surg Am 1991;16:1125–9.

45. Gordon L, Levinsohn DG, Moore SV, et al. The Sauvé-Kapandji procedure for the treatment of post-traumatic distal radioulnar problems. Hand Clin 1991;7(2):397–403.

46. Schneider LH, Imbriglia JE. Radio-ulnar joint fusion for distal radio-ulnar joint instability. Hand Clin 1991;7:391–5.

47. Condamine JL, Lebreton L, Aubriot JH. L'intervention de Sauvé-Kapadji. Ann Chir Main 1992;11:27–39 [in French].

48. Millroy P, Coleman S, Ivers R. The Sauvé-Kapandji operation. Technique and results. J Hand Surg Br 1992;17:411–4.

49. Johnson RK, Shewsbury MM. The pronator quadratus in motions and stabilization of the radius and ulna at the distal radioulnar joint. J Hand Surg 1976;1:205–9.

50. Gabl M, Zimmermann R, Angermann P, et al. The interosseous membrane and its influence on the distal radioulnar joint. J Hand Surg Br 1998;23:179–82.

51. Ward LD, Ambrose CG, Masson MV, et al. The role of the distal radioulnar ligaments, interosseous membrane, and joint capsule in distal radioulnar joint capsule in distal radioulnar joint stability. J Hand Surg Am 2000;25:341–51.

52. McConkey MO, Schwab TD, Travlos A, et al. Quantification of pronator quadratus contribution to isometric pronation torque of the forearm. J Hand Surg Am 2009;34:1612–7.

53. Stuart PR. Pronator quadratus revisited. J Hand Surg Br 1996;21(6):714–22.

54. Daecke W, Martini AK, Schneider S, et al. Amount of ulnar resection is a predictive factor for ulnar instability problems after the Sauve-Kapandji procedure: a retrospective study of 44 patients followed for 1-3 years. Acta Orthop 2006;77:290–7.

55. Noble J, Arafa M. Stabilisation of distal ulna alter excessive Darrach's procedure. Hand 1983;15(1):70–2.

56. Breen TF, Jupiter JB. Extensor carpi ulnaris and flexor carpi ulnaris tenodesis of the unstable distal ulna. J Hand Surg Am 1989;14:612–7.

57. Lamey DM, Fernandez DL. Results of the modified Sauvé-Kapandji procedure in the treatment of chronic posttraumatic derangement of the distal radioulnar joint. J Bone Joint Surg Am 1998;80:1758–69.

58. Lees VC, Scheker LR. The radiological demonstration of dynamic ulnar impingement. J Hand Surg Br 1997;22:448–50.

59. McKee MD, Richards RR. Dynamic radio-ulnar convergence after the Darrach procedure. J Bone Joint Surg Br 1996;78:413–8.

60. Shaaban H, Giakas G, Bolton M, et al. The distal radioulnar joint as a load-bearing mechanism: a biomechanical study. J Hand Surg Am 2004;29:85–95.

Periprosthetic Bone Resorption and Sigmoid Notch Erosion Around Ulnar Head Implants: A Concern?

Guillaume Herzberg, MD, PhD

KEYWORDS

- Radius sigmoid notch erosion • Radioulnar impingement
- Ulnar head implants • Bone resorption

Fifteen years have elapsed between the first description of ulnar impingement syndrome after ulnar head resection[1] and the first report of a series of ulnar head implants.[2] During this period, studies by Hagert[3] and Lees and Scheker[4] made it progressively obvious that both the Darrach and Sauvé-Kapandji operations (or any of their variants) were "destabilizing procedures" in relation to the whole forearm. Dynamic radioulnar impingement after the Darrach or Sauvé-Kapandji procedures for arthritic distal radioulnar joint (DRUJ) is unavoidable because of the loss of the solid ulnar head support.[4] Because what is lacking is a solid ulnar head volume, none of the many soft tissue stabilizing procedures that have been proposed for unstable symptomatic Darrach or Sauvé-Kapandji operations can solve the problem. Ulnar impingement syndrome after a Darrach or Sauvé-Kapandji procedure is symptomatic in about 20% to 30% of cases.[5] Metallic ulnar head implants,[2,6–12] total DRUJ prostheses,[13,14] and Achilles allograft interposition[15,16] have been proposed to treat symptomatic ulnar impingement syndrome. Substantial improvements have been reported after each of these salvage surgical procedures.[2,11,14,15] For this reason, metallic ulnar head implants have been proposed not only to solve symptomatic impingement after Darrach or Sauvé-Kapandji procedures but also to prevent such an impingement when treating arthritic DRUJ. The largest reports of metallic ulnar head implant[2,11] have noted sigmoid fossa remodeling and bone resorption at the prosthesis collar. These phenomena have been said to stabilize with time[2,11] but no detailed data have been provided about this stabilization. This article prospectively analyzes a series of ulnar head implants with special reference to sigmoid erosion and bone resorption at the prosthesis collar.

METHODS

Between 2003 and 2008, 17 ulnar head implants were implanted by one surgeon in 17 patients (13 female and 4 male) in one wrist surgery center after careful informed consent for a new procedure. The indications for ulnar head implants were symptomatic radioulnar impingement after a Darrach procedure in four patients, and after a Sauvé-Kapandji procedure in two patients. Primary indications of ulnar head implants were chosen in five rheumatoid wrists, four distal radius malunions, one distal ulna giant cell tumor, and one primary osteoarthritis with fourth and fifth extensor tendon ruptures. Several associated surgical procedures were performed: three radiolunate fusions and one radioscapholunate fusion in the five patients with rheumatoid wrists, one radiolunate fusion and two radioscapholunate fusions in the four patients with distal radius malunions, and side-to-side fourth and fifth extensor tendon repairs in the patient with primary osteoarthritis. All patients

Division of Hand and Upper Extremity Orthopaedic Surgery, Herriot Hospital and Claude Bernard University, 5 Place Arsonval, 69437 Lyon Cedex 03, France
E-mail address: guillaume.herzberg@chu-lyon.fr

Hand Clin 26 (2010) 573–577
doi:10.1016/j.hcl.2010.08.001
0749-0712/10/$ — see front matter © 2010 Elsevier Inc. All rights reserved.

Table 1
Specific clinical criteria used in this study

	0	5	10	15	20
Pain with forearm rotation	Severe	Important	Moderate	Climatic or heavy use	None
Impairment of rotational forearm function	Severe	Important	Moderate	Minimal	None
Active arc of forearm rotation	0–39°	40°–79°	80°–119°	120°–160°	>160°
Grip strength (% of contralateral)	0–24	25–49	50–74	75–99	100

were included in a prospective nonrandomized study with follow-up clinical and radiologic studies at 6 weeks, 6 months, and every year after the operation. Clinical criteria are described in **Table 1**. The results were expressed in percentages and considered as excellent (≥85%); good (≥70%); fair (≥50%); or poor (<50%). Clinical stability of the implant or snapping with forearm rotation was carefully followed. Subjective results were also recorded (much better, better, unchanged, worse, or much worse).

Radiologically, special attention was provided to radial sigmoid notch erosion and bone resorption around the collar of the prosthesis. A bone resorption index (BRI) was defined as the ratio between the length of the pericollar bone resorption and the length of the stem of the implant (**Fig. 1**). A radial sigmoid notch erosion index (SEI) was defined as the ratio between the width of the distal radius at the level of the DRUJ and the width of the implant at the same level (**Fig. 2**).

Among the first 11 patients, there were two re-operations. One patient had an early (sixth postoperative month) implant removal because of persistent ulnar pain and implant snapping despite satisfactory radiographs. The indication had been an arthritic DRUJ complicating a distal radius articular malunion; a radiolunate fusion was

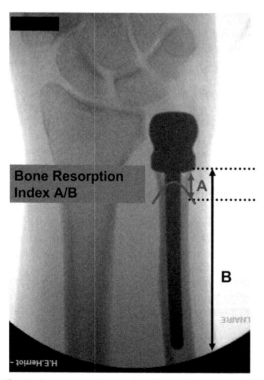

Fig. 1. Bone resorption index (A and B expressed in millimeters).

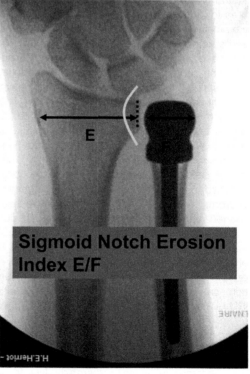

Fig. 2. Radial sigmoid notch erosion index (E and F expressed in millimeters).

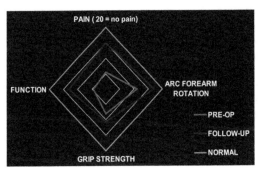

Fig. 3. Clinical results.

performed in conjunction with the ulnar head implant. The radiolunate fusion healed but the patient requested the implant to be removed because of the snapping. A very difficult removal of the implant (a bone window had to be made into the ulnar diaphysis all along the stem of the implant) was done and associated with a modified Breen and Jupiter[17,18] operation. Another patient had a dorsal shortening capsuloplasty 6 months after the implant operation for dorsal clinical and radiological implant instability.

Ten patients had more than 24 months of follow-up (average, 36 months; minimum, 25 months; and maximum, 63 months). These 10 patients provide the basis of the current clinical and radiologic results.

RESULTS
Clinical Results

Visual analog scale pain with forearm rotation improved from 7.4 preoperatively to 2 postoperatively.

The pronosupination pain score improved from 5.5 points preoperatively to 15 points postoperatively. The rotational forearm function score improved from 4.5 points preoperatively to 13 points postoperatively. Postoperative pronosupination arc was 146° compared with 108° preoperatively. The pronosupination score improved from 11 points preoperatively to 17 points postoperatively. The grip strength score improved from 8 points preoperatively to 10.5 points postoperatively. Overall, the specific score used in this study improved from an average of 36.5 preoperatively to 68.9 postoperatively with significant improvement of pain, function, and arc of forearm rotation and modest improvement of grip strength (**Fig. 3**). There were four excellent, two good, two fair, and two poor results. Subjectively, four patients were much better, five were better, and one was unchanged. One 30-year-old active female rheumatoid patient was of special interest because she had a radiolunate fusion combined with a Darrach procedure on her right dominant side (11 years of follow-up) that could be compared (**Fig. 4**) with a radiolunate fusion combined with an ulnar head implant on the opposite side (3 years follow-up). Despite the absence of postoperative complication or reoperation on either wrist, her clinical score as expressed previously was 66% (fair) at the "Darrach side" compared with 88% (excellent) at the "implant side." There was painful radioulnar impingement with forearm rotation at the "Darrach side" compared with a smooth painless forearm rotation at the

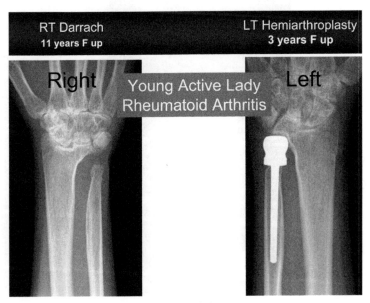

Fig. 4. Radiographs of patient #4 (see text for clinical results).

"implant side" and a much higher patient satisfaction.

Radiological Results

Bone resorption around the collar of the prosthesis was observed in 90% of the 10 cases at the average follow-up of 36 months. At follow-up, the BRI averaged 7% (0%–18%). Examples of minimal, average, and maximum resorption are shown in **Fig. 5**. It was interesting to follow the BRI with time. The BRI increased significantly during the first postoperative year, and then remained stable until maximum follow-up in each patient (**Fig. 6**).

Radial sigmoid notch erosion opposite to the implant was observed in 30% of the cases at the average follow-up of 36 months. The SEI decreased from an average of 1.9 (1.5–2.6) on the immediate postoperative radiographs to an average of 1.8 (1.4–2.6) on the follow-up radiographs.

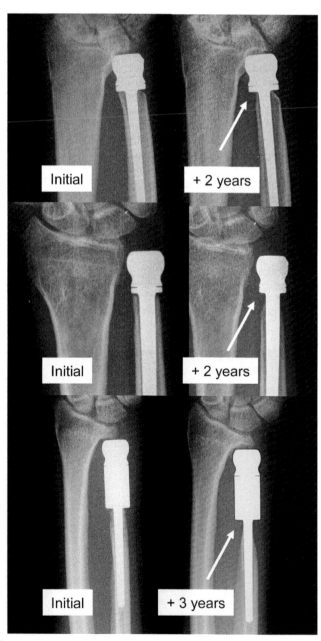

Fig. 5. Examples of bone resorption.

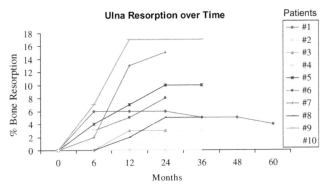

Fig. 6. Stabilization of the bone resorption index with time.

DISCUSSION

The current clinical results of this prospective single center, single surgeon study are in accordance with the clinical results of the two largest reports of ulnar head implants.[2,11] The special radiologic study about bone resorption around the collar of the prosthesis confirmed this almost constant phenomenon[2,11] related to stress shielding around the implant. It could be demonstrated on this small sample of patients who were followed prospectively that the bone resorption occurred within the first postoperative year, then stabilized from 1 year to an average follow-up of 3 years. Such a detailed radiologic study about periprosthetic bone resorption has not been reported to date. Similarly, a detailed follow-up of radial sigmoid notch erosion opposite to the implant showed that the erosion was minimal at an average of 3 years. Further studies are needed to determine if this minimal erosion stands the test of a long-term follow-up and if it is related to the size of the implant.

REFERENCES

1. Bell MJ, Hill RJ, McMurtry RY. Ulnar impingement syndrome. J Bone Joint Surg Br 1985;67(1):126–9.
2. Van Schoonhoven J, Fernandez DL, Bowers WH, et al. Salvage of failed resection arthroplasties of the distal radio-ulnar joint using a new ulnar head prosthesis. J Hand Surg Am 2000;25:438–46.
3. Hagert CG. The distal radioulnar joint in relation to the whole forearm. Clin Orthop 1992;275:56–64.
4. Lees VC, Scheker LR. The radiological demonstration of dynamic ulnar impingement. J Hand Surg Br 1997;22(4):448–50.
5. George MS, Stern PJ. The Sauve Kapandji procedure and the Darrach procedure for distal radio-ulnar joint dysfunction after Colles fracture. J Hand Surg Br 2004;29:608–13.
6. Berger RA, Cooney WP. Use of an ulnar head endoprosthesis for treatment of an unstable distal ulnar resection: review of mechanics, indications, and surgical techniques. Hand Clin 2005;21:603–20.
7. Cooney WP, Berger RA. DRUJ implant arthroplasty. J Am Soc Surg Hand 2005;5:217–31.
8. Fernandez DL. Treatment of failed SK procedures with a spherical ulnar head prosthesis. Clin Orthop 2006;445:100–7.
9. Kopylov P, Tagil M. Distal radio ulnar joint replacement. Tech Hand Up Extrem Surg 2007;11:109–14.
10. Sauder DJ, King GJ. Hemiarthroplasty of the distal ulna with an eccentric prosthesis. Tech Hand Up Extrem Surg 2007;11:115–20.
11. Willis AA, Berger RA, Cooney WP. Arthroplasty of the DRUJ using a new ulnar head endoprosthesis: preliminary report. J Hand Surg Am 2007;32:177–89.
12. Shipley NY, Bowers WH. Ulnar head implant arthroplasty. An intermediate term review of 1 surgeon's experience. Tech Hand Up Extrem Surg 2009; 13:160–4.
13. Laurentin-Perez LA, Scheker LR. A study of functional outcomes following implantation of a total DRU joint prosthesis. J Hand Surg Br 2008;33:18–28.
14. Scheker LR. Implant arthroplasty for the distal radio-ulnar joint. J Hand Surg Am 2008;33:1639–44.
15. Sotereanos DG. An allograft salvage technique for failure of the Darrach procedure: a report of 4 cases. J Hand Surg Br 2002;27:317–21.
16. Greenberg JA, Sotereanos DG. Achilles allograft interposition for failed Darrach distal ulna resections. Tech Hand Up Extrem Surg 2008;12:121–5.
17. Breen TF, Jupiter JB. Extensor carpi ulnaris and flexor carpi ulnaris tenodesis of the unstable distal ulna. J Hand Surg Am 1989;14:612–7.
18. Breen TF, Jupiter JB. Tenodesis of the chronically unstable distal ulna. Hand Clin 1991;7(2):355–63.

The Management of Congenital and Acquired Problems of the Distal Radioulnar Joint in Children

Tamir Pritsch, MD[a], Steven L. Moran, MD[b,c],*

KEYWORDS

- Distal radioulnar joint • Madelung deformity
- Forearm physeal arrest • Osteochondromatosis

Pain in the ulnar aspect of the pediatric wrist is an uncommon problem; however, when pain does occur it is usually the result of antecedent bony trauma or an underlying skeletal abnormality. Developmental skeletal deformities that may lead to ulnar-sided wrist pain include Madelung deformity, physeal arrest, and osteochondromatosis. It is important for the clinician to be able to identify these entities within the pediatric wrist in order to make the appropriate diagnosis and plan for surgical intervention to prevent ongoing damage to the distal radioulnar joint (DRUJ). The purpose of this article is to review the etiology, clinical presentation, and treatment strategies for the management of these unique problems that can affect the pediatric and adolescent DRUJ.

DEVELOPMENT OF THE DRUJ

A distinguishing feature in man and hominoid primates is the complete separation of the DRUJ from the radiocarpal joint by means of a fibrous articular disk. This separation has allowed for longitudinal forearm rotation independent from the movement at the carpal joint, and has developed over the course of evolution;

however, a component of this separation of forearm and carpus still occurs during early fetal development.[1]

Cihak[2] has shown, based on the study of 62 embryonic and fetal specimens, that early in development the ulnar styloid is in contact with the triquetrum. As the fetus grows there is differential growth between the radius and ulna, resulting in the gradual recession of the ulna from the carpus.[3] Recession is found to occur early in development when the fetal crown-rump length is only 45 mm. During the ulna's recession, there is the simultaneous formation of the ulnocarpal ligaments and triangular fibrocartilage complex (TFCC).[1,4] This developmental process of differential growth between radius and ulna may account for the variations seen within the geometry of the DRUJ as well as the final position of the ulnar head in reference to the radius and carpus.[5] It is of interest that in Cihak's studies the lunate was found initially to be positioned between the radius and ulna before its migration distal into the proximal carpal row; this more proximal position of the lunate is often seen in Madelung syndrome, and may suggest a failure of lunate

[a] Department of Orthopedics, 143 Avalon Cove Circle NW, Rochester, MN 55901, USA
[b] Division of Plastic Surgery, Department of Surgery, Mayo Clinic, 200 First Street SW, Rochester, MN 55905, USA
[c] Division of Hand Surgery, Department of Orthopaedic Surgery, Mayo Clinic, 200 First Street SW, Rochester, MN 55905, USA
* Corresponding author. Division of Hand Surgery, Department of Orthopaedic Surgery, Mayo Clinic, 200 First Street SW, Rochester, MN 55905.
E-mail address: moran.steven@mayo.edu

Hand Clin 26 (2010) 579–591
doi:10.1016/j.hcl.2010.06.001
0749-0712/10/$ — see front matter © 2010 Elsevier Inc. All rights reserved.

migration early within DRUJ development (**Fig. 1**).[2]

MADELUNG DEFORMITY

The Madelung deformity is usually identified radiographically in adolescent or preadolescent females presenting with pain at the wrist and DRUJ, and a prominent ulnar head. Madelung[6] originally described the deformity in 1878, without the aid of radiographs. Later radiographic studies would show that the pathology is due to abnormal physeal growth within the radius, resulting in increased palmar and ulnar tilt of its articular surface with shortening and sometimes bowing of the radial shaft (see **Fig. 1**). The carpus is often palmarly and ulnarly subluxated. The lunate is often displaced proximally, lying between the radius and ulna, as originally identified in Cihak's[2] anatomic studies. The ulna, which is thought to develop normally during this disease process, is prominent dorsally, resulting in symptoms of impaction as well as instability and subluxation of the DRUJ.[7,8]

The incidence of Madelung deformity is not clear, and in one series it comprised 7 of 1000 consecutive congenital upper limb anomalies.[9] It is 4 times more common in females, and most patients present with bilateral changes.[10] The genetic basis for the development of the deformity is still under investigation, but studies have found that the deformity has been strongly linked to mutations in the short homeobox-containing gene (SHOX). Abnormalities within this gene can also result in Leri-Weill dyschondrosteosis (an autosomal dominant syndrome with 50% penetrance). Leri-Weill syndrome results in patients with a short stature, Madelung-like wrist deformity, and shortening of the middle segment of the extremities (mesomelia).[10–13] Several studies have suggested that Madelung deformity is never found in isolation and is always a component of Leri-Weill dyschondrosteosis[10,14]; this claim is still debatable, as others, including Madelung, have described the wrist deformity occurring as an isolated condition.[7,15,16]

Several conditions may mimic the Madelung deformity radiographically. These diagnoses can include osteochondromatosis, radial physeal arrest, achondroplasia, Turner syndrome, nail-patella syndrome, sepsis, and previous trauma (**Fig. 2**). Genetic evaluation and computed tomography scans may be required to rule out these possible diagnoses.

Pathophysiology

According to observations by Vickers and Nielsen,[17] deformity within the distal radius is due to a combination of both bony and ligamentous abnormalities. The dyschondrosteosis in the distal radius most commonly occupies the volar ulnar third of the physis; this area of physeal pathology not only fails to grow but also acts as a tether. The dyschondrosteotic lesion can also be located centrally or dorsally, which results in carpal triangularization without visible deformity, or a reverse Madelung deformity with dorsal angulation of the distal radius, respectively; however, these presentations are less common. An abnormal thick volar ligament, the so-called Vickers ligament, has been identified in several cases, and appears to strongly tether the lunate in a proximal position between or below the radius and ulna; it may also cause thinning of the radial epiphysis by maintaining a constant compression force against the radius.[17] Others have suggested that the abnormal ligament may merely represent a soft tissue compensatory response secondary to the progressive loss of support of the lunate facet, and the need to support the carpus.[18]

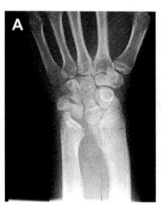

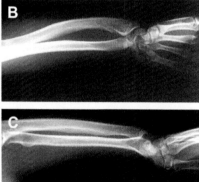

Fig. 1. (*A–C*) Anteroposterior (AP) and lateral radiographs of a 14-year-old girl with the Madelung deformity of both wrists. The Madelung deformity is thought to develop because of abnormal physeal growth within the radius. The typical deformities within the wrist are depicted, including increased ulnar and palmar tilt of the radial articular surface. The radius is shortened with frequent bowing of the shaft. Note how the lunate (*A*), appears to be pulled proximal and ulnar.

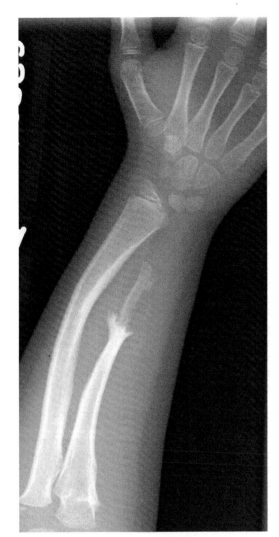

Fig. 2. AP radiographs of the forearm of a 6-year-old girl showing a "Madelung type" deformity. The radius in this patient is bowed and there is the appearance of a physeal tether at the ulnar aspect of the radial physis; however, this forearm deformity is the result of osteomyelitis of the ulnar shaft, which has resulted in an ulnar nonunion and a premature closure of the ulnar physis.

Presentation

Madelung deformity is not apparent in infancy or early childhood, and most commonly becomes apparent between the ages of 6 and 13 years.[19–21] Radiographic abnormalities can be identified at an early age at the distal radius, but the growth spurt in late childhood in conjunction with a premature fusion across the physis usually results in the clinical manifestation of the deformity (**Fig. 3**).[17] Forearms in patients with the Madelung deformity are typically short and stout with evidence of bowing.

The most visible deformity is the prominence of the ulnar head dorsally. Despite the clinical appearance at this early age, there may be minimal functional impairment. Symptomatic patients often complain of ulnar-sided wrist pain and limitation of motion, primarily supination.[17,22,23] Pain is suspected to be caused by the mechanical derangement of the DRUJ, and by degenerative changes in the opposing articular surfaces of the lunate and the radius.[24] A painful deformity is an acceptable indication for surgical treatment. In addition, many patients dislike the appearance of their forearm caused by the radial bowing and the dorsally prominent ulna, and are interested in a cosmetic improvement.[25] Recommending a prophylactic surgical treatment, in the absence of pain, is still controversial, as the correlation between the degree of the deformity and the severity of pain or the alteration in range of motion has not been clearly demonstrated.

Radiographic Findings

Several investigators have defined the radiographic abnormalities involved in the Madelung deformity (see **Fig. 1**).[26,27] Abnormalities seen within the radius include dorsal and ulnar curvature, decreased length, triangularization and unequal growth of the distal radial epiphysis, premature fusion of the medial half of the radial epiphysis, a localized area of lucency along the ulnar border of the radius, osteophyte formation along the inferior ulnar part of the radius, and ulnar and palmar angulation of the distal radial articular surface. Changes involving the ulna include dorsal subluxation, enlargement and distortion of the ulnar head, and decreased length. Changes involving the carpal bones include wedging between the radius and ulna and a triangular configuration of the lunate bone (**Fig. 4**).

Treatment

The goal of treatment is to decrease pain, improve range of motion, and achieve an improved cosmetic result. Patients with significant growth remaining often benefit from resection of the physeal lesion (physiolysis) and division of the abnormal volar ligament tethering the lunate to the radius. Vickers and Nielsen[17] reported satisfactory results using this procedure with significant improvement in pain, range of motion, and improvement of the radiographic deformity. Regardless of the growth potential, releasing the Vickers ligament was reported to have a beneficial effect on pain and resulted in some degree of carpal reduction (**Fig. 5**).[28,29] An osteotomy of the distal radius is probably preferable over

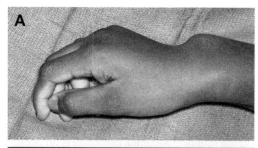

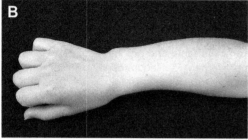

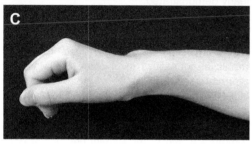

Fig. 3. (*A*) Clinical manifestation of Madelung deformity in an 11-year-old girl, showing significant prominence of the ulnar head. (*B, C*) A 16-year-old girl with a less severe deformity; the forearm shows clinical evidence of bowing and there is dorsal prominence of ulnar head.

a physiolysis for correction of deformities of patients with limited remaining growth. The group of Carter and Ezaki[28–30] has popularized the biplanar dome osteotomy, which in comparison to wedge osteotomies makes the correction of 3-dimensional deformities easier. Of the 26 wrists treated with dome osteotomies in their series, 2 patients hand concomitant ulnar epiphysiodesis, 2 patients had simultaneous ulnar shortening, and 4 patients elected to undergo ulnar shortening later on. All patients in their series reported reduction in pain and improvement in the appearance of the wrist. These investigators also demonstrated a significant improvement in pronation and supination, and no loss of overall wrist motion (**Fig. 6**). Alternatively, a dorsal closing wedge osteotomy with ulnar shortening or an opening wedge osteotomy of the radius can be performed, addressing the positive ulnar variance, which for many patients is a significant source of pain.[31,32]

Murphy and colleagues[31] reported pain relief and improved cosmesis in all 11 patients in their series of open wedge osteotomy of the distal radius; however, there was no improvement in range of motion or grip strength. In addition, dos Reis and colleagues[32] treated 25 wrists with Madelung deformity with wedge subtraction osteotomy of the radius and shortening of the ulna; they demonstrated a significant improvement in grip strength and range of motion. Eighty percent of their patients reported improvement in pain, and 88% were satisfied with the appearance. The use of the Ilizarov distraction osteogenesis technique, which facilitates gradual correction in multiple planes, has also been reported, with significant improvement in pain and range of motion, and 100% patient satisfaction rate with the functional and cosmetic results.[33] For mild deformity localized to the ulnar aspect of the wrist, ulnar shortening alone has been recommended.[34] Finally, for those patients who present late with evidence of DRUJ arthritis, ulnar head resection or a Suave-Kapandji procedure have been recommended. These techniques can be combined with some form of correction of the radial deformity if warranted.[25,35]

DISTAL FOREARM PHYSEAL ARRESTS

Traumatic or infectious insults to the growth plates of the distal radius and ulna may lead to growth arrest and consequently disrupt their normal development, causing increasing deformity and subsequent incongruity and instability of the radiocarpal and distal radioulnar joints. Risk factors for the development of physeal arrest include high-energy injuries involving the growth plate, repetitive compression loading across the physis (as is seen in young gymnasts), multiple traumatic reduction attempts of displaced physeal fractures, and late attempt at physeal fracture reduction (**Fig. 7**).[36,37]

Physeal Development

The distal radial epiphysis normally appears between 0.5 and 2.3 years in boys and 0.4 and 1.7 years in girls.[38] Initially the epiphysis has a straight appearance, but progresses to a triangular shape as the radial styloid elongates with advancing skeletal maturity. The secondary center of ossification for the distal ulna appears at about age 7 years. Similar to the radius, the ulnar styloid appears with the adolescent growth spurt. It also becomes more elongated during the process of physeal closure. On average, the distal ulnar physis closes at age 16 in girls and age 17 in boys, whereas the distal radial physis closes on

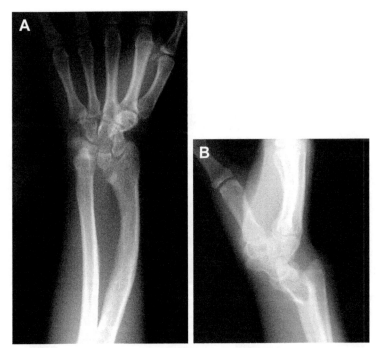

Fig. 4. (*A*) Additional radiographic features seen in Madelung deformity include significant proximal and ulnar translation of the lunate resulting in a wedge appearance of the carpus as well as a triangular appearance of the lunate. (*B*) Lateral radiographs show evidence of significant palmar translation of the carpus.

average 6 months later.[39] The distal radial and ulnar physes contribute approximately 75% to 80% of the growth of the forearm and 40% of the growth of the upper extremity,[40] and their synchronized growth maintains the integrity and functionality of the DRUJ.

Etiology

Injury to either ulnar or radial physis is possible following forearm fractures. Distal radius fractures are among the most common pediatric injuries, comprising 20% to 35% of all childhood fractures.[41,42] One-third of pediatric distal radius fractures involve the growth plate, which makes it the second most common long bone physeal injury following phalangeal fractures.[43,44] Surprisingly, whereas up to two-thirds of children have been reported to have growth retardation after distal radius fractures,[45] significant growth disturbances following physeal fractures of the distal radius are relatively rare. Cannata and colleagues[46] reported the long-term outcomes on 157 distal radius physeal fractures and found only 4.4% incidence of clinically significant radial shortening. Similarly, Bae and Waters[47] reported a 4% incidence of clinical or radiographic evidence of growth arrest among 290 displaced

distal radius physeal fractures. Growth arrest following nonphyseal distal radius fractures has been documented in only a few case reports in the English literature. Most reports attribute the growth arrest to an associated crash injury to the physis (Salter Harris type V injury), which cannot be appreciated radiographically in the acute setting.[48] Premature physeal closure was also reported in teenage girl gymnasts, and was considered to be related to chronic physeal injury.[49] Fractures to the distal ulnar physis are less common and account for only about 5% of all physeal injuries; however, in contrast to distal radius physeal fractures, the frequency of growth arrest is much higher.[46,50]

Current treatment recommendations for displaced physeal fractures of either the distal radius or ulna include attempts at atraumatic reduction within 7 days of injury. If closed reduction is not possible then open reduction should be attempted. If fixation is required then the surgeon must avoid creating an iatrogenic physeal injury. In such cases surgical screws should not, if possible, cross the physeal plate. Placement of small-diameter smooth pins perpendicular to the central physeal region for a short periods of time is the authors' preferred method of treatment. Pin size, the presence of

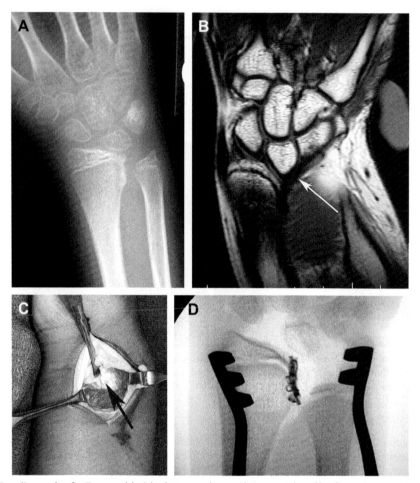

Fig. 5. (*A*) AP radiograph of a 7-year-old girl whose mother and sister each suffer from the Madelung deformity. The radiograph shows evidence of an early physeal tether at the ulnar aspect of the radial physis. (*B*) T1-weighted magnetic resonance (MR) coronal image of the wrist verifying the presence of the Vickers ligament, a thickening of the short radiolunate ligament, within this patient (*white arrow*). (*C, D*) Surgical procedure. At the time of surgery the ligament is identified below the pronator and then divided with the scalpel. (*C*) The cut ligament is shown (*black arrow*), while the Freerer elevator points to the articular surface of the lunate. Following division of the Vickers ligament, a physiolysis is performed at the site of physeal arrest. Fat from the forearm is used as an interpositional graft to prevent retethering of the physis. (*D*) Placement of a radio-opaque sponge to mark the site of the physiolysis.

threads, pin location in the physis, and angle of pin penetration may all play a role in the probability of developing an iatrogenic physeal injury.[51]

Finally, infection can lead to partial or complete physeal arrest. Physeal insults can result secondary to neonatal sepsis or osteomyelitis. In these cases the growth plate is destroyed by the infection, resulting in replacement of the affected component with a bony bridge following the resolution of the infection.[52,53]

Pathophysiology

The physeal arrest is caused by the replacement of the physis with a bony bridge, binding the epiphysis to the metaphysis, and preventing further growth in this zone. The overall effect depends on multiple factors including the size of the bridge, its location, and the amount of growth remaining. A peripheral bridge forms a pivot point causing angular deformity, whereas a central bridge causes tenting of the physis, shortening, and joint deformity. Some small bridges can break down spontaneously, so as not to cause long-term complications.[54]

Significant radial growth arrest may lead to a relative ulnar overgrowth and altered radial inclination, resulting in abnormal wrist mechanics, ulnocarpal impaction, possible triangular fibrocartilage tears, and DRUJ instability. Growth arrest

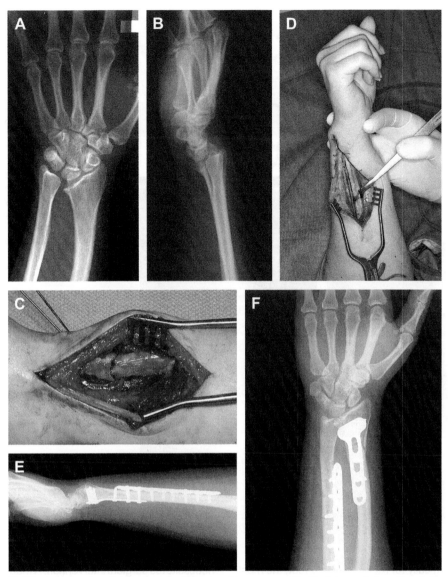

Fig. 6. (*A, B*) AP and lateral radiographs of a 26-year-old woman with Madelung deformity of the wrist. The patient underwent a simultaneous radial dome osteotomy (*C*) to correct the palmar and ulnar tilt of the radial articular surface in conjunction with an ulnar shortening procedure (*D*). (*E, F*) Final AP and lateral radiographs showing the correction in dorsal translocation of the ulna. The patient had significant improvement in pain and range of motion of the forearm following the procedure.

in the ulna may result in DRUJ pathology and an ulnar minus variant. In addition, ulnar growth arrest may cause a tethering effect on the distal radius, leading to radial bowing and soft tissue contracture of the ulnar side of the wrist.[37,55]

In a biomechanical cadaveric study of the effect of radial deformity on the kinematics of the DRUJ, radial shortening was found to cause the greatest disturbance in the kinematics of the TFCC; dorsal angulation with decreased radial inclination resulted in intermediate changes to the TFCC, whereas dorsal displacement of the radius alone produced minimal changes.[56] The size of a clinically significant radioulnar length discrepancy was only anecdotally studied, and is inconsistent between different series. In a long-term follow-up study of distal forearm physeal fractures, Cannata and colleagues[46] found radial shortening of greater than 1 cm produced evidence of significant clinical problems. In a series of 30 patients

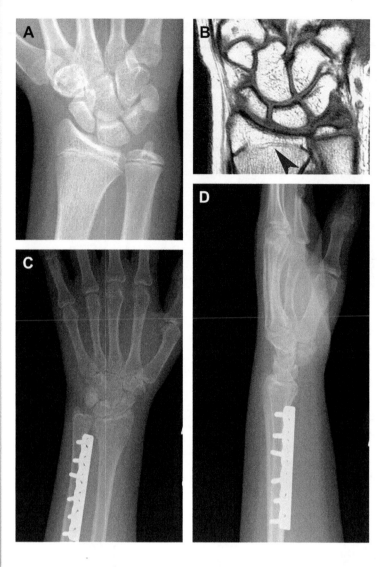

Fig. 7. (*A–D*). A 13-year-old female gymnast who presented with significant ulnar-sided wrist pain with clinical findings of ulnar impaction. (*A, B*) AP and lateral radiographs revealed an ulnar positive variance with premature closure of the radial physis. (*C*) T1-weighted MR image of the wrist showing premature closure of the central portion of the radial physis (*black arrow*). Treatment consisted of ulnar shortening osteotomy with concomitant closure of the ulnar physis. (*D*) AP radiograph 6 months after surgery, showing closure of the ulnar physis and an ulnar neutral variance across the wrist. The patient was able to return to gymnastics.

treated surgically for radial growth arrest, the most frequent preoperative impairments were activity-related pain and loss of wrist motion, particularly pro-supination; TFCC tears were identified in 13 cases.[37]

Treatment

Ideally, physeal arrest of the distal radius will be discovered early, before the consequences of unbalanced growth develop; therefore, it is imperative that the hand surgeon perform close follow-up until skeletal maturity in cases of known physeal injury. Close patient follow-up allows early detection, and consequently simpler and more successful surgical solutions.[54] A small area of growth arrest in a patient near skeletal maturity may be clinically inconsequential; however, a large area of arrest in a patient with marked growth remaining

necessitates surgical intervention. A magnetic resonance imaging scan can map the area of arrest. If the area is less than 45% of the physis a bar resection can be attempted, which may restore radial growth and prevent future problems. If the osseous bridge is larger than 45% of the physis, bar resection is unlikely to be successful, and thus other surgical procedures should be considered.[57]

To achieve the goals of a radiocarpal joint with neutral ulnar variance, a stable DRUJ and TFCC, and improved radial inclination and volar tilt, Waters and colleagues[37] have proposed the use of the following treatment algorithm. To attain neutral ulnar variance, patients with minor ulnar overgrowth and some remaining radial growth underwent ulnar epiphysiodesis. Patients with more severe ulnar overgrowth underwent ulnar shortening osteotomy. Ulnar shortening and ulnar epiphysiodesis can be combined if significant ulnar growth remains. To achieve appropriate radial inclination and tilt, patients with progressive radial deformity but greater than 10° of inclination were treated with completion of radial epiphysiodesis, in patients with less than 10° of inclination an open wedge osteotomy was performed, and both procedures were combined if significant growth remained. Peripheral TFCC tears were repaired, and radial tears were debrided. In cases of DRUJ instability, repair of the TFCC stabilized the joint in most cases.[37] Radial growth arrests that result in a significant shortening or a complex 3-dimensional deformity are surgically challenging and may necessitate a different approach. Considerably shortening the ulna to compensate for a significant radial shortening can result in a cosmetically shortened forearm.

In such cases of significant radial deficiency, radial lengthening can be considered. Radial lengthening can be performed acutely using an open wedge technique or a z-lengthening and an autogenous bone graft,[58,59] or in a gradual fashion using callus distraction with external unilateral or Ilizarov ring fixator.[53,60] Hove and Engesaeter[58] reported on 6 patients with radial growth arrest who underwent radial lengthening with an iliac bone graft, or ulnar shortening, depending on the severity of the deformity. Postoperatively all patients were pain free, and range of motion was 93% to 100% of the contralateral side. Recently, a successful use of the Taylor spatial frame has been described to correct radial deficiency. Seybold and colleagues[60] were able to achieve an anatomic reduction and improvement in range of motion using this device.

OSTEOCHONDROMAS OF THE FOREARM BONES

Multiple osteochondromata, also called multiple exostoses, is a disorder of enchondral bone growth, manifested by abnormal metaphyseal bone prominences capped with cartilage. Lesions are often accompanied by a defective metaphyseal remodeling and asymmetric retardation of longitudinal bone growth, which is probably secondary to their proximity to the growth plate.[61] Malignant degeneration of the lesion, most commonly resulting in the development of chondrosarcomas, have been reported to occur in approximately 1% of affected patients.[62] In the forearm, osteochondromas most frequently affect the distal ulna followed by the distal radius.[63] These lesions can often result in growth arrest, DRUJ involvement, and occasional instability.

Presentation and Natural History

Osteochondromas are often discovered after the age of 2 to 3 years. Osteochondromas continue to enlarge with skeletal growth and can lead to weakness, functional impairment, and cosmetic deformity. The lesions stop enlarging once skeletal maturity is reached.[63,64] Deformities of the forearm are seen in 30% to 60% of patients with this disorder. A common feature of forearm involvement is bowing of the radius and a relative shortening of the ulna (**Fig. 8**). Additional abnormalities include increased ulnar tilt of the distal epiphysis of the radius, ulnar deviation of the hand, progressive ulnarward translocation of the carpus, and dislocation of the proximal radial head.[63,65]

Noonan and colleagues[66] reported on the natural history of patients with multiple osteochondromatosis involving the forearm. Objective measurements demonstrated restriction of elbow, forearm, and wrist range of motion, as well as functional limitations. Surprisingly, 88% of involved forearms were pain free, and only 13% of patients reported that they were limited in any way in the performance of their jobs. Moreover, radiographic evaluation demonstrated arthritic changes in only 3 of the 77 involved forearms. Similarly, Arms and colleagues[67] found that such patients do subjectively well after skeletal maturity, without having undergone aggressive surgical interventions.

Other investigators have recommended early aggressive surgery to prevent or reduce the progression of the deformity, and limit possible functional impairment in the upper extremity.[62,63,65,68] Although the functional beneficial effect of surgery is controversial, there is an agreement that cosmetic appearance can often be improved, and that a significant percentage of skeletally mature patients who did not have surgical correction are unhappy with the appearance of their upper extremities.[62,65,66]

Treatment

Several surgical interventions for the management of forearm deformities have been described, including simple excision of the osteochondroma, acute or gradual ulnar lengthening, corrective radial osteotomy, hemiepiphyseal stapling of the distal radius, the Sauve-Kapandji procedure, and creation of one-bone forearm.[61,63,69–71]

The most common surgical procedure performed is simple excision. Some investigators claim that osteochondromata should be excised as soon as it becomes clear that growth patterns of the involved bones are being altered,[61] whereas others have observed that the excision of the

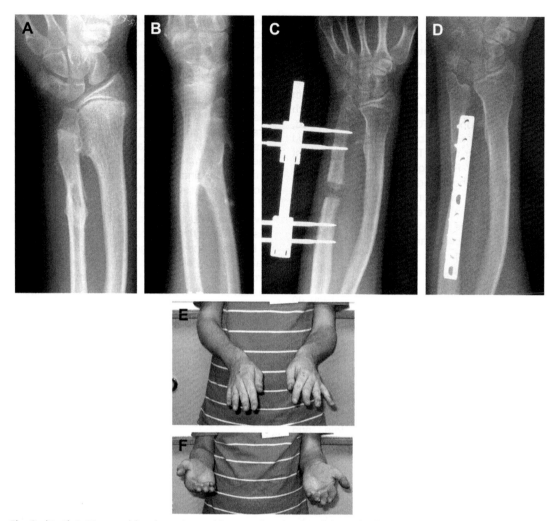

Fig. 8. (*A–F*) A 16-year-old male patient with osteochondroma of the right distal radius and ulna. (*A, B*) Involvement of the ulna has resulted in ulnar negative variance, limitations in pronation and supination, as well as ulnar-sided wrist pain. (*C, D*) Treatment consists in resection of osteochondromas in addition to distraction lengthening of the ulna. Following distraction, a plate was applied to the ulna. (*D*) AP radiograph of the wrist 1 year after the procedure. (*E, F*) Pain has improved, and pronation and supination are equivalent to contralateral side.

lesion was not effective in controlling the progression of the deformity.[63] Several investigators have found simple excision to improve the range of motion of the forearm.[70,71] Masada and colleagues[69] reported excellent functional results after simple excision of osteochondroma as long as the procedure was limited to those with relative radial shortening secondary to distal osteochondroma of the radius. Conversely, Wood and colleagues[65] demonstrated improved cosmesis after simple excision in 4 patients, but only minimal improvement in rotation of the forearm. Ishikawa and colleagues[72] found that the location of the exostosis affects the results of a simple excision in correcting the forearm deformity; in their series, forearms with solitary distal ulnar lesions were

significantly better corrected after excision, compared with forearms with lesions in both the distal ulna and ulnar aspect of the distal radius.[72] Other indications for excision of osteochondromas include the presence of pain (usually the result of repeated external trauma to the prominence), and rapid enlargement with radiographic changes suggestive of malignant transformation.

When simple excision of an osteochondroma is undertaken, all of the cartilage cap must be removed while avoiding violation of the physis. In addition, the margins of the surgical incision should be palpated for adjacent bumps, which may not be visible on radiographs because of their cartilaginous nature. Bone wax can be employed for any persistent bony bleeding.

The treatment of the hypoplastic ulna can include lengthening in a gradual or an acute fashion (see **Fig. 8**). Lengthening the ulna not only addresses the negative variance but also decreases the tethering effect on the ulnar side of the radial physis, and consequently decreases the abnormally increased radial articular angle.[61] Pritchett[73] reported a series of 10 forearms with multiple exostoses that were treated with ulnar lengthening, and demonstrated improved cosmesis and improved radial deviation in all cases; forearm rotation and radial head stability were improved in most cases. Conversely, Fogel and colleagues[63] reported only occasional correction of the ulnar drift of the distal radius following ulnar lengthening; they also found that ulnar lengthening alone did not result in a significant improvement of forearm rotation, and that the relative shortening of the ulna had recurred. For this reason, overdistraction of the ulna is not considered detrimental if the child is still growing. Similarly, Shin and colleagues[70] did not find a discernible clinical or radiographic improvement with ulnar lengthening. Akita and colleagues[71] also reported that ulnar lengthening could be associated with multiple complications, including nonunions, fracture, and temporary radial nerve paresis.

Radial deformities can be approached directly with hemiepiphyseal stapling, or with shortening osteotomy. Hemiepiphysiodesis of the distal radius can correct the radial articular angle, but has less effect on radioulnar length discrepancy, and is considered to be a good adjunctive treatment to improve the radiocarpal relationship.[62,63] Radial shortening was only rarely used to equalize the radioulnar length discrepancy, and very often is undesirable, as the involved forearm is already shorter than the contralateral forearm.[61]

All of the aforementioned procedures may be used in conjunction with one another to achieve a balanced forearm. Matsubara and colleagues reported satisfactory results with resection of the exostosis, correction of the radial deformity, and gradual lengthening of the ulna using an external fixator. Significant improvement in pro-supination was shown in 6 of their 7 patients. Waters and colleagues[59] reported the return of good function and improved radiographs with the use of acute equalization of the radioulnar length in 17 forearms with multiple exostoses. In this report Waters and colleagues tailored their treatment for each deformity, using different combinations of exostosis excision, ulnar lengthening, radial osteotomy, and hemiepiphyseal stapling. Lastly, Shin and colleagues[70] reported improved wrist stability, and better forearm range of motion following a Sauvé-Kapandji procedure combined with simple excision of the osteochondromas; mean supination increased by 11.2°, pronation by 21.4°, and the radial articular angle and carpal slip also improved.

SUMMARY

Developmental abnormalities in the ulnar aspect of the wrist are rare, but when they do occur they can result in impairment to the DRUJ, producing ulnar-sided wrist pain. Indications for surgery include ongoing pain, decreased function, and a desire for an improved cosmetic appearance of the wrist. Because of the low incidence of these disorders, the current literature includes mostly small retrospective series with a low level of evidence. Further multicenter prospective series will be required to determine the value of prophylactic surgery and the benefits of one surgical procedure over another. Until that time, the surgeon should make every effort to identify these problems early and tailor any surgical intervention to the child's functional needs.

REFERENCES

1. Louis DS, Jebson PJ. The evolution of the distal radio-ulnar joint. Hand Clin 1998;14:155–9.
2. Cihak R. Ontogenesis of the skeleton and intrinsic muscles of the human hand and foot. Folia Morphol 1972;21:228–31.
3. Beatty E. Tissue differentiation of the upper extremity. In: Gupta A, Kay SP, Scheker LR, editors. The growing hand. 1st edition. Philadelphia: Mosby; 2000. p. 33–8.
4. Kauer JM. The distal radioulnar joint: anatomical and functional considerations. Clin Orthop Relat Res 1992;275:5–13.
5. DeSmet L. Ulnar variance: fact and fiction review article. Acta Orthop Belg 1994;60:1–9.
6. Madelung O. Die spontane subluxation der hand nach norne. Archiv fur Klinische Chirurgie 1878;23:395–412 [in German].
7. Golding JS, Blackburne JS. Madelung's disease of the wrist and dyschondrosteosis. J Bone Joint Surg Br 1976;58(3):350–2.
8. Vickers D. Madelung's deformity. In: Cooney WP, Linschied RL, Dobyns JH, editors. The wrist—diagnosis and operative treatment. 1st edition. St Louis (MO): Mosby; 1998. p. 966–81.
9. Ogino T, Minami A, Fukuda K, et al. Congenital anomalies of the upper limb among the Japanese in Sapporo. J Hand Surg Br 1986;11:364–71.
10. Herdman RC, Langer LO, Good RA. Dyschondrosteosis. The most common cause of Madelung's deformity. J Pediatr 1966;68:432–41.

11. Dawe C, Wynne-Davies R, Fulford GE. Clinical variation in dyschondrosteosis. A report on 13 individuals in 8 families. J Bone Joint Surg Br 1982;64: 377–81.

12. Belin V, Cusin V, Viot G, et al. SHOX mutations in dyschondrosteosis (Leri-Weill syndrome). Nat Genet 1998;19(1):67–9.

13. Shears DJ, Vassal HJ, Goodman FR, et al. Mutation and deletion of the pseudoautosomal gene SHOX cause Leri-Weill dyschondrosteosis. Nat Genet 1998;19(1):70–3.

14. Zebala LP, Manske PR, Goldfarb CA. Madelung's deformity: a spectrum of presentation. J Hand Surg Am 2007;32(9):1393–401.

15. Felman AH, Kirkpatrick JA Jr. Madelung's deformity: observations in 17 patients. Radiology 1969;93: 1037–42.

16. Plafki C, Luetke A, Willburger RE, et al. Bilateral Madelung's deformity without signs of dyschondrosteosis within five generations in a European family—case report and review of the literature. Arch Orthop Trauma Surg 2000;120:114–7.

17. Vickers D, Nielsen G. Madelung deformity: surgical prophylaxis (physiolysis) during the late growth period by resection of the dyschondrosteosis lesion. J Hand Surg Br 1992;17:401–7.

18. Ty JM, James MA. Failure of differentiation: part II (arthrogryposis, camptodactyly, clinodactyly, Madelung deformity, trigger finger, and trigger thumb). Hand Clin 2009;25:195–213.

19. Cook PA, Yu JS, Wiand W, et al. Madelung deformity in skeletally immature patients: morphologic assessment using radiography, CT, and MRI. J Comput Assist Tomogr 1996;20:505–11.

20. Schmidt-Rohlfing B, Schwobel B, Pauschert R, et al. Madelung deformity: clinical features, therapy, results. J Pediatr Orthop B 2001;10:344–8.

21. Thomas RD, Fairhurst JJ, Clarke NM. Madelung's deformity masquerading as a bone tumour. Skeletal Radiol 1993;22:329–31.

22. Fagg PS. Wrist pain in Madelung's deformity of dyschondrosteosis. J Hand Surg Br 1988;13(1): 11–5.

23. Bruno RJ, Blank JE, Ruby LK, et al. Treatment of Madelung's deformity in adults by ulna reduction osteotomy. J Hand Surg Am 2003;28(3):421–6.

24. Henry A, Thorburn MJ. Madelung's deformity. A clinical and cytogenetic study. J Bone Joint Surg Br 1967;49:66–73.

25. James MA, Bender M. Madelung's deformity. In: Green DP, Hotchkiss RN, Pederson WC, et al, editors. Greens operative hand surgery. 5th edition. Philadelphia: Elsevier; 2005. p. 1484–9.

26. Dennenberg M, Anton JI, Spiegel MB. Madelung's deformity. Consideration of its roentgenological diagnostic criteria. Am J Roentgenol 1939;42: 671–6.

27. Langer LO. Dyschondrosteosis, a hereditable bone dysplasia with characteristic roentgenographic features. Am J Roentgenol 1965;95: 178–88.

28. Carter PR, Ezaki M. Madelung's deformity: surgical correction through the anterior approach. Hand Clin 2000;16(4):713–21.

29. Harley BJ, Carter PR, Ezaki M. Volar surgical correction of Madelung's deformity. Tech Hand Up Extrem Surg 2002;6(1):30–5.

30. Harley BJ, Brown C, Cummings K, et al. Volar ligament release and distal radius dome osteotomy for correction of Madelung's deformity. J Hand Surg Am 2006;31:1499–506.

31. Murphy MS, Linscheid RL, Dobyns JH, et al. Radial opening wedge osteotomy in Madelung's deformity. J Hand Surg Am 1996;21(6):1035–44.

32. Dos Reis FB, Katchburian MV, Faloppa F, et al. Osteotomy for the radius and ulna for the Madelung deformity. J Bone Joint Surg Br 1998;80(5):817–24.

33. Houshian S, Schrøder HA, Weeth R. Correction of Madelung's deformity by the Ilizarov technique. J Bone Joint Surg Br 2004;86(4):536–40.

34. Ranawat CS, DeFiore J, Straub LR. Madelung's deformity. An end-result study of surgical treatment. J Bone Joint Surg Am 1975;57:772–5.

35. DeSmet L, Fabry G. Treatment of Madelung's deformity by Kapandji's procedure and osteotomy of the radius. J Pediatr Orthop B 1993;2:96–8.

36. Aminian A, Schoenecker PL. Premature closure of the distal radial physis after fracture of the distal radial metaphysic. J Pediatr Orthop 1995;15:495–8.

37. Waters PM, Bae DS, Montgomery KD. Surgical management of posttraumatic distal radial growth arrest in adolescents. J Pediatr Orthop 2002;22: 717–24.

38. Garn SM, Rohmann CG, Silverman FN. Radiographic standards for postnatal ossification and tooth calcification. Med Radiogr Photogr 1967;43: 45–66.

39. Mino DE, Palmer AK, Levinsohn EM. Radiography and computerized tomography in the diagnosis of incongruity of the distal radio-ulnar joint. A prospective study. J Bone Joint Surg Am 1985; 67:247–52.

40. Ogden JA, Beall JK, Conlogue GJ, et al. Radiology of postnatal skeletal development. IV. Distal radius and ulna. Skeletal Radiol 1981;6:255–66.

41. Cheng JC, Shen WY. Limb fracture pattern in different age groups: a study of 3350 children. J Orthop Trauma 1993;7:15–22.

42. Worlock P, Stower M. Fracture patterns in Nottingham children. J Pediatr Orthop 1986;6:656–60.

43. Mann DC, Rajmaira S. Distribution of physeal and nonphyseal fractures of long bones in children aged 0 to 16 years. J Pediatr Orthop 1990;10: 713–6.

44. Peterson HA, Madhok R, Benson JT, et al. Physeal fractures: PART 1. Epidemiology in Olmsted County, Minnesota, 1979–1988. J Pediatr Orthop 1994;14: 423–30.

45. Aitken AP. Further observations on the fractured distal radial epiphysis. J Bone Joint Surg 1935; 17:922–7.

46. Cannata G, De Maio F, Mancini F, et al. Physeal fractures of the distal radius and ulna: long-term prognosis. J Orthop Trauma 2003;17(3):172–9.

47. Bae DS, Waters PM. Pediatric distal radius fractures and triangular fibrocartilage complex injuries. Hand Clin 2006;22(1):43–53.

48. Tang CW, Robert MK, Skaggs DL. Growth arrest of the distal radius following a metaphyseal fracture: case report and review of the literature. J Pediatr Orthop B 2002;11:89–92.

49. Talat AR, Sanderson PL, DeSmet L, et al. The gymnast's wrist: acquired positive ulnar variance following epiphyseal injury. J Hand Surg Br 1992; 17(6):678–81.

50. Nelson OA, Buchanan JR, Harrison CS. Distal ulnar growth arrest. J Hand Surg Am 1984;9(2):164–70.

51. Boyden EM, Peterson HA. Partial premature closure of the distal radial physis associated with Kirschner wire fixation. Orthopedics 1991;14:585–8.

52. Peters W, Irving J, Letts M. Long term effects of neonatal bone and joint infection on adjacent growth plates. J Pediatr Orthop 1992;12:806–10.

53. Price CT, Mills WL. Radial lengthening for septic growth arrest. J Pediatr Orthop 1983;3:88–91.

54. Vickers D. Growth plate injuries. In: Cooney WP, Linschied RL, Dobyns JH, editors. The wrist—diagnosis and operative treatment. 1st edition. St Louis (MO): Mosby; 1998. p. 982–90.

55. Golz RJ, Grogan DP, Greene TL, et al. Distal ulnar physeal injury. J Pediatr Orthop 1991;11(3):318–25.

56. Adams BD. Effects of radial deformity on distal radioulnar joint mechanics. J Hand Surg Am 1993;18: 492–8.

57. Waters PM, Mih AD. Fractures of the distal radius and ulna. In: Beaty JH, Kasser JR, editors. Rockwood and Wilkins' fractures in children. 6th edition. Philadelphia: Lippincott Williams & Wilkins (LWW); 2006. p. 337–98.

58. Hove LM, Engesaeter LB. Corrective osteotomies after injuries of the distal radial physis in children. J Hand Surg Br 1997;22(6):699–704.

59. Waters PM, Van Heest AE, Emans J. Acute forearm lengthening. J Pediatr Orthop 1997;17(4):444–9.

60. Seybold D, Geßmann J, Muhr G, et al. Deformity correction with the Taylor spatial frame after growth arrest of the distal radius. Acta Orthop 2008;79:571–5.

61. Peterson HA. Deformities and problems of the wrist in children with multiple hereditary osteochondroma. In: Coony WP, Linscheid RL, Dobyns JH, editors. The wrist—diagnosis and operative treatment. 1st edition. St. Louis (MO): Mosby; 1998. p. 991–1001.

62. Peterson HA. Multiple hereditary osteochondromata. Clin Orthop Relat Res 1989;239:222–30.

63. Fogel GR, McElfresh EC, Peterson HA, et al. Management of deformities of the forearm in multiple hereditary osteochondromas. J Bone Joint Surg Am 1984;66(5):670–80.

64. Bock GW, Reed MH. Forearm deformities in multiple cartilaginous exostoses. Skeletal Radiol 1991;20(7): 483–6.

65. Wood VE, Sauser D, Mudge D. The treatment of hereditary multiple exostosis of the upper extremity. J Hand Surg Am 1985;10:505–13.

66. Noonan KJ, Levenda A, Sned J, et al. Evaluation of the forearm in untreated adult subjects with multiple hereditary osteochondromatosis. J Bone Joint Surg Am 2002;84:397–403.

67. Arms DM, Stecker WB, Manske PR, et al. Management of forearm deformity in multiple hereditary osteochondromatosis. J Pediatr Orthop 1997;17:450–4.

68. Burgess C, Cates H. Deformities of the forearm in patients who have multiple cartilaginous exostoses. J Bone Joint Surg Am 1993;75:13–8.

69. Masada K, Tsuyuguchi Y, Kawai H, et al. Operations for forearm deformity caused by multiple osteochondromas. J Bone Joint Surg Br 1989; 71:24–9.

70. Shin EK, John NF, Lawrence JF. Treatment of multiple hereditary osteochondromas of the forearm in children. A study of surgical procedures. J Bone Joint Surg Br 2006;88:255–60.

71. Akita S, Murase T, Yonenobu K, et al. Long-term results of surgery for forearm deformities in patients with multiple cartilaginous exostoses. J Bone Joint Surg Am 2007;89(9):1993–9.

72. Ishikawa J, Kato H, Fujioka F, et al. Tumor location affects the results of simple excision for multiple osteochondromas in the forearm. J Bone Joint Surg Am 2007;89(6):1238–47.

73. Pritchett JW. Lengthening the ulna in patients with hereditary multiple exostosis. J Bone Joint Surg Br 1986;68:561–5.

Index

Note: Page numbers of article titles are in **boldface** type.

A

Adams-Berger procedure. See *Radioulnar ligament(s), volar and dorsal, reconstruction of.*

Allograft interposition procedure, in failed surgery of distal radioulnar joint, 534

Arthroplasty, Darrach resection, in arthrosis of distal radioulnar joint, 530–531
    radioulnar impingement after, 573
    ulnar head implants after, 573

Arthroscopic repair, and open repair, of triangular fibrocartilage complex, **485–494**

Arthroscopy, of distal radioulnar joint, 477

B

Bone resorption, periprosthetic, and sigmoid notch erosion around ulnar head implants, **573–577**

Bone resorption index, 574
    ulnar head implants and, 576, 577

C

Capsulorrhaphy procedure, extensor retinaculum, in chronic instability of distal radioulnar joint, 522–523

Capsulotomy, radio-ulno-carpal, 482–483
    radioulnar, 483

CT, of distal radioulnar joint, 469–471
    device for use with, 469, 470

D

Darrach resection arthroplasty, in arthrosis of distal radioulnar joint, 530–531
    radioulnar impingement after, 573
    ulnar head implants after, 573

E

Essex-Lopresti injury, 508–509

Extensor carpi ulnaris, distal radioulnar joint and, 465

Extensor retinaculum capsulorrhaphy procedure, in chronic instability of distal radioulnar joint, 522–523

F

Forearm, anteroposterior view of, in full pronation, 459–460
    distal, physeal arrests of, 582–587
        etiology of, 583–584

        pathophysiology of, 584–586
        treatment of, 586–587
    osteochondromas of, 587–589
        presentation and natural history of, 587
        treatment of, 587–589
    whole, lateral view of distal radioulnar joint and, 460

Forearm procedure, one-bone, in failed surgery of distal radioulnar joint, 538–539

G

Galeazzi fracture, 506–508
    treatment of, 506–508

I

Interosseous membrane, anatomy and biomechanics of, 543, 544
    distal radioulnar joint and, 504
    injuries to, management of, **543–548**
    treatment of, 543–547
        passage of graft in, 545, 547

L

Leri-Weill dyschondrosteosis, Madelung deformity and, 580

Linscheid-Hui procedure, in chronic instability of distal radioulnar joint, 523

M

Madelung deformity, 580–582
    and Leri-Weill dyschondrosteosis, 580
    conditions mimicking, 580, 581
    pathophysiology of, 580
    presentation of, 581, 582
    radiographic findings in, 581, 582
    treatment of, 581–582, 584, 585

MRI, of distal radioulnar joint, 471–473

Multiple exostoses. See *Osteochondromas, of forearm.*

O

One-bone forearm procedure, in failed surgery of distal radioulnar joint, 538–539

Osseous reconstruction, autograft, in failed surgery of distal radioulnar joint, 534–535

Osteochondromas, of forearm, 587–589
    presentation and natural history of, 587
    treatment of, 587–589

Hand Clin 26 (2010) 593–595
doi:10.1016/S0749-0712(10)00078-8
0749-0712/10/$ – see front matter © 2010 Elsevier Inc. All rights reserved.

hand.theclinics.com

United States Postal Service

Statement of Ownership, Management, and Circulation
(All Periodicals Publications Except Requestor Publications)

1. Publication Title	2. Publication Number	3. Filing Date
Hand Clinics	0 0 0 - 7 0 9 9	9/15/10

4. Issue Frequency	5. Number of Issues Published Annually	6. Annual Subscription Price
Feb, May, Aug, Nov	4	$316.00

7. Complete Mailing Address of Known Office of Publication (Not printer) (Street, city, county, state, and ZIP+4®)	Contact Person
Elsevier Inc.	Stephen Bushing
360 Park Avenue South	Telephone (Include area code)
New York, NY 10010-1710	215-239-3688

8. Complete Mailing Address of Headquarters or General Business Office of Publisher (Not printer)

Elsevier Inc., 360 Park Avenue South, New York, NY 10010-1710

9. Full Names and Complete Mailing Addresses of Publisher, Editor, and Managing Editor (Do not leave blank)

Publisher (Name and complete mailing address)

Kim Murphy, Elsevier, Inc., 1600 John F. Kennedy Blvd. Suite 1800, Philadelphia, PA 19103-2899

Editor (Name and complete mailing address)

Deb Dellapena, Elsevier, Inc., 1600 John F. Kennedy Blvd. Suite 1800, Philadelphia, PA 19103-2899

Managing Editor (Name and complete mailing address)

Barbara Cohen-Kligerman, Elsevier, Inc., 1600 John F. Kennedy Blvd. Suite 1800, Philadelphia, PA 19103-2899

10. Owner (Do not leave blank. If the publication is owned by a corporation, give the name and address of the corporation immediately followed by the names and addresses of all stockholders owning or holding 1 percent or more of the total amount of stock. If not owned by a corporation, give the names and addresses of the individual owners. If owned by a partnership or other unincorporated firm, give its name and address as well as those of each individual owner. If the publication is published by a nonprofit organization, give its name and address.)

Full Name	Complete Mailing Address
Wholly owned subsidiary of	4520 East-West Highway
Reed/Elsevier, US holdings	Bethesda, MD 20814

11. Known Bondholders, Mortgagees, and Other Security Holders Owning or Holding 1 Percent or More of Total Amount of Bonds, Mortgages, or Other Securities. If none, check box ☐ None

Full Name	Complete Mailing Address
N/A	

12. Tax Status (For completion by nonprofit organizations authorized to mail at nonprofit rates) (Check one)
The purpose, function, and nonprofit status of this organization and the exempt status for federal income tax purposes:
☐ Has Not Changed During Preceding 12 Months
☐ Has Changed During Preceding 12 Months (Publisher must submit explanation of change with this statement)

PS Form 3526, September 2007 (Page 1 of 3 (Instructions Page 3)) PSN 7530-01-000-9931 PRIVACY NOTICE: See our Privacy policy in www.usps.com

---

13. Publication Title	14. Issue Date for Circulation Data Below
Hand Clinics	August 2010

15. Extent and Nature of Circulation		Average No. Copies Each Issue During Preceding 12 Months	No. Copies of Single Issue Published Nearest to Filing Date
a. Total Number of Copies (Net press run)		1858	1834
b. Paid Circulation (By Mail and Outside the Mail)	(1) Mailed Outside-County Paid Subscriptions Stated on PS Form 3541. (Include paid distribution above nominal rate, advertiser's proof copies, and exchange copies)	1029	976
	(2) Mailed In-County Paid Subscriptions Stated on PS Form 3541 (Include paid distribution above nominal rate, advertiser's proof copies, and exchange copies)		
	(3) Paid Distribution Outside the Mails Including Sales Through Dealers and Carriers, Street Vendors, Counter Sales, and Other Paid Distribution Outside USPS®	357	362
	(4) Paid Distribution by Other Classes Mailed Through the USPS (e.g. First-Class Mail®)		
c. Total Paid Distribution (Sum of 15b (1), (2), (3), and (4))	▶	1386	1338
d. Free or Nominal Rate Distribution (By Mail and Outside the Mail)	(1) Free or Nominal Rate Outside-County Copies Included on PS Form 3541	64	25
	(2) Free or Nominal Rate In-County Copies Included on PS Form 3541		
	(3) Free or Nominal Rate Copies Mailed at Other Classes Through the USPS (e.g. First-Class Mail)		
	(4) Free or Nominal Rate Distribution Outside the Mail (Carriers or other means)		
e. Total Free or Nominal Rate Distribution (Sum of 15d (1), (2), (3) and (4))	▶	64	25
f. Total Distribution (Sum of 15c and 15e)	▶	1450	1363
g. Copies not Distributed (See instructions to publishers #4 (page #3))	▶	408	471
h. Total (Sum of 15f and g)	▶	1858	1834
i. Percent Paid (15c divided by 15f times 100)		95.59%	98.17%

16. Publication of Statement of Ownership

☐ If the publication is a general publication, publication of this statement is required. Will be printed in the November 2010 issue of this publication.   ☐ Publication not required

17. Signature and Title of Editor, Publisher, Business Manager, or Owner		Date
[signature] Stephen R. Bushing – Fulfillment/Inventory Specialist		September 15, 2010

I certify that all information furnished on this form is true and complete. I understand that anyone who furnishes false or misleading information on this form or who omits material or information requested on the form may be subject to criminal sanctions (including fines and imprisonment) and/or civil sanctions (including civil penalties).

PS Form 3526, September 2007 (Page 2 of 3)

Moving?

Make sure your subscription moves with you!

To notify us of your new address, find your **Clinics Account Number** (located on your mailing label above your name), and contact customer service at:

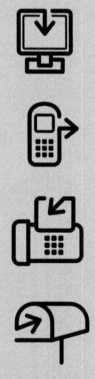

Email: journalscustomerservice-usa@elsevier.com

800-654-2452 (subscribers in the U.S. & Canada)
314-447-8871 (subscribers outside of the U.S. & Canada)

Fax number: 314-447-8029

Elsevier Health Sciences Division
Subscription Customer Service
3251 Riverport Lane
Maryland Heights, MO 63043

*To ensure uninterrupted delivery of your subscription, please notify us at least 4 weeks in advance of move.

Printed and bound by CPI Group (UK) Ltd, Croydon, CR0 4YY

03/10/2024

01040344-0020